DANCE INJURIES
Their prevention and care

DANIEL D. ARNHEIM, D.P.E., F.A.C.S.M., A.T.C.

Professor, California State University, Long Beach, California

THIRD EDITION

A DANCE HORIZONS BOOK
Princeton Book Company, Publishers
Princeton, NJ 08534

Index by Judith Hancock
Typesetting by TypeHouse of Pennington
Printed by Versa Press

A Dance Horizons Book
Princeton Book Company, Publishers
POB 57
Pennington, NJ 08534

Library of Congress Catalog Card Number: 90-053353

ISBN 0-87127-146-X

Preface

It is a source of great pleasure to learn that reader interest in the first and second editions of *Dance Injuries: Their Prevention and Care* has been sufficient to warrant a third edition. The first and second editions pioneered an area relatively new to the dance profession. At that time, little concrete information was available on injuries specifically occurring to dancers, and there was some question as to whether such a text would be accepted by the profession.

Since the second edition, serious interest seems to have developed about injury prevention and care, as is attested to by the increased number of articles and amount of research appearing on these topics. Dance kinesiology is increasingly being accepted among dancers, with attention to both typical and atypical body movements. Dancers also have become much more sophisticated in understanding the scientific ramifications of the human body engaged in dance. By its expanded content and scope, this edition reflects dancers' increased knowledge of kinesiology and heightened interest in the medical aspects of dance injuries.

As in previous editions, *Dance Injuries: Their Prevention and Care* is divided into five parts, each providing a logical sequence of information to help the dancer intelligently understand the many aspects of physical disabilities stemming from the dance environment. Part I, "Concerns and Directions," introduces the reader to dance injuries, what the state of the art is, and the current practices taking place. Part II, "Why Dance Injuries?" discusses the dancer's body, its susceptibility to injury, and specifically the stresses imposed on the dancer's body by engaging in dance. Part III, "Major Factors in Injury Prevention," presents the ways in which injuries may be prevented through proper conditioning, nutrition, and dealing with psychological factors inherent in dance.

Part IV, "Principles of Injury Care," gives the bases for evaluating and managing musculoskeletal problems most common to dancers. Cold and heat therapy are discussed in depth, along with massage and reconditioning exercises. The principles of using protective and supportive materials that can be easily employed by dancers are also discussed. Special therapeutic methods commonly used by dancers, such as the manipulative sciences, rolfing, and reflex methods such as shiatsu or acupressure, are included.

Part V, "Musculoskeletal Conditions Common to Dance," uses the information imparted in earlier chapters to thoroughly explain the most prevalent injuries occurring in dance. Chapters in this section are devoted to understanding compression injuries (including contusions), friction problems, strains, and joints and skeletal problems (including sprains, dislocations, and fractures).

Dance Injuries: Their Prevention and Care has extensive illustrations, including charts and tables, drawings, and photographs. Step-by-step instructions are given for practical application of therapeutic methods and exercises.

Many thanks are extended to Diane Defenderfer for her suggestions and photographic assistance. Diane is the model for all the new photographs. She is a former soloist for the Frankfurt and Los Angeles ballets and provided expertise in proper and faulty ballet positions throughout the text. Diane currently is ballet instructor at The University of California, Irvine, and the director and owner of the Studio Du Corps (using Pilates methodology), 151 Kalmus, Suite 63, Costa Mesa, California 92626. Thanks are also extended to photographer David M. Lee.

Daniel D. Arnheim

Contents

IV

PRINCIPLES OF INJURY CARE

V

MUSCULOSKELETAL CONDITIONS COMMON TO DANCE: THEIR PREVENTION, RECOGNITION, EVALUATION, AND MANAGEMENT

I

CONCERNS AND DIRECTIONS

Dance, especially theatrical or concert dance, often places extreme and unusual demands on the body. With an ever increasing number of individuals entering the ranks of aspiring dancers, there is a vital need for paying special attention to the prevention of disabling injury and the ability to properly manage these injuries once they present themselves. Attention must be drawn to the performer and the dance educator as well as the choreographer and the stage manager. Each of these specialists must become aware of the limits of the human body and the scientific principles associated with effective conditioning and environmental manipulation that provide optimum defense against the physiological and psychological stresses imposed by a particular dance form. These specialists must also be cognizant of the injury or the symptoms of injury that are beyond their scope of knowledge and/or experience and that may require professional care. It is to these ends that **Dance Injuries: Their Prevention and Care** is dedicated.

1

What is the concern?

Dance is an art form in which the body is the instrument of expression. When it comes to seeking movement perfection, no physical endeavor can compare with dance. Few sports can compare with dance in terms of time and energy expended, and the physical, mental and emotional demands that are made. In seeking maximum expression of style and technique, dancers often exceed their physical capacities. The result is an injury that may be temporary or, in many cases, permanent. A severe injury could exclude the dancer from future participation in dance. Lack of knowledge of the body's limitations and how to properly care for it often causes the dancer needless incapacitation and inactive time.

In general, dance can be divided into two categories: (1) recreational or social and (2) concert or theatrical. Under the theater and concert umbrella fall the dance forms of ballet, modern, jazz, ethnic, and character, all of which have particular characteristics and peculiarities that may produce physical trauma. In recent years, there has been a steady increase of interest in these dance forms. This current interest must in some ways be attributed to the influence of the media, the increased support of local cultural groups throughout the nation, and the burgeoning college and university programs leading to advanced degrees in dance. Of the vast number of individuals interested in dance performance, few are accepted into dance companies, and even fewer reach national acclaim.

Musculoskeletal injuries are thought to be one of the main reasons why many potentially outstanding dancers are prevented from reaching the top of their chosen field. This is understandable when one considers that a usual weekly work schedule for a dancer includes 9 hours in class, 26 hours in rehearsal, and 8 to 12 hours in performance, over a 6 day period.[21] It has often been said that "one day of practice missed, the dancer can tell; two days missed, the audience can tell." With this adage in mind, the dancer will very often try to dance through an injury rather than take the time out to properly

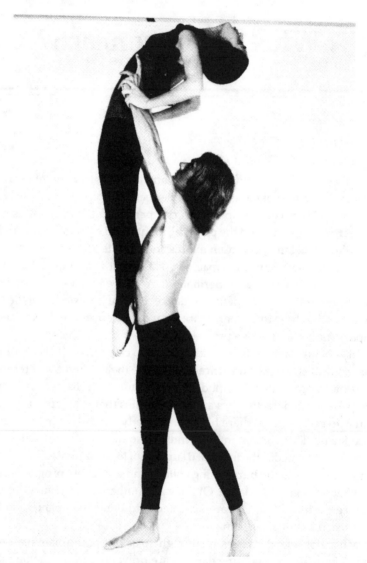

Fig. 1-1. Few activities compare with dance in terms of the demands placed on the body.

care for it or to obtain a professional opinion as to its severity. In the process of continuing to dance while injured, the dancer avoids the ailing part, thereby placing increased stress, tension, and strain on other body parts, which may lead to additional injuries. Every dancer's injury is the responsibility of all who are associated with dance: the dancer, choreographer, teacher, and stage manager.

Many other factors added to a fatiguing schedule can predispose the dancer to injury. Some of these are poor conditioning, improper warm-up and cool-down, faulty technique, and anatomical variations.[23] The feet, ankles, lower legs, knees, hips, and lower back, in general, have the highest incidence of injury by the performance of dance.

Each dance form places its own particular stress on the body. In ballet, precise movements are performed, often in contradiction to more typical

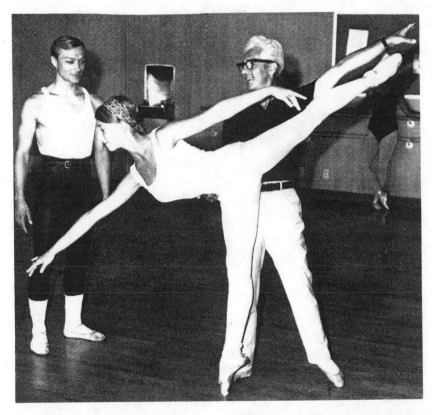

Fig. 1-2. Ballet can place great stress on the body. At California State University, Long Beach Summer School of Dance, Alfredo Corvino teaches ballet technique.

body movements, that can cause many injuries to the feet, legs, and hips. In contrast, modern dance (Fig. 1-1) is performed by strong muscular contractions and releases of the trunk with movements that are commonly more exaggerated and angular than those associated with ballet. Jazz, on the other hand, may require quick and ballistic movements, whereas ethnic dance— such as ceremonial, religious, or social dances that are representative of a specific ethnic group—is highly variable as to the stresses imposed on the body.

Until recently, dancers have sadly neglected to learn proper prevention and management of their injuries (Fig. 1-2). This has been partially due to a failure to accept and practice known scientific principles for fear that science and art were incompatible. With the advent of dance kinesiology, the dance profession is beginning to accept the science of movement as it plays a positive and integral role in dance by enhancing aesthetics and preventing injury.

2

The basic four

Human beings were concerned about traumatic injuries and disease long before recorded time. Primitive tribesmen would perish if an incapacitating injury or disease made them unable to forage for food or defend themselves against hostile enemies. From a basic need for survival emerged the healing modalities of heat, massage, and therapeutic exercise. The soothing relief of hot springs or warm sun rays became common sources of therapy for early people. Through the ages, primitive and more sophisticated cultures alike found that rubbing the body in a certain manner would bring about healing responses and that certain types of active movement could help an injured or diseased person return more quickly to normalcy. Soon, specialists in healing methods became important officials of early cultures. The primary duty of these medicine men and women, or shamans, was to prevent illness through rituals and to treat the ill and incapacitated by the use of selected therapeutic techniques. A comparison of past and current practices shows that not much has changed in healing approaches; the only real change has come about in the degree of sophistication in the care of injuries.

Four major factors are highly important in assisting the natural healing process. These key factors are: preventive conditioning, immediate injury care, follow-up care, and supportive techniques.

PREVENTIVE CONDITIONING

In the last few years, preventive conditioning has become increasingly important to the dance and sports worlds. Instead of being most concerned after an injury has occurred we now emphasize prevention of injuries "before the fact." In dance, injuries can be decreased by the employment of proper conditioning methods. Preventive conditioning strives to obtain a balance between strength, flexibility, and stamina. To prevent injury there must be a generally high level of strength throughout the body, with more strength available than is required to minimally execute a given skill. However, overspecialization of strength development must be avoided. In other words, strength should not be developed just for a particular skill but should be acquired so that prime movers and assisters are equally balanced in strength with opposing muscles. The old saying that "a person is only as strong as his or her weakest link" can certainly be applied to muscular strength.

Although it should never be developed at the expense of good muscle tone, flexibility is a major factor in the prevention of injury. Despite the ballet dancers' apparent leg flexibility, for example, they characteristically have a tight iliotibial band that may lead to knee and hip pain. Dancers often attempt to exceed anatomical limitations in their desire to become more flexible, and in doing so they often neglect strength in a specific area, which eventually may lead to joint disease.

When preventive conditioning is considered, endurance cannot be underestimated. Staying power, or stamina, means the ability to withstand fatigue and engage in arduous activity over a long period. It is of the utmost importance for the dancer engaged in a performance that demands a high level of precision and energy output to remain as fresh at the end of the performance as at the beginning.

The concept of preventive conditioning is as important for the time a dancer is actually performing as it is for rehearsing or studying. Those involved in high-intensity physical activities are becoming more cognizant of the fact that the physical training that prepares them for a particular dance is not enough to sustain them throughout a dance season, as the patterns of movement themselves do not normally maintain the level of conditioning required for optimum performance. Consequently, there is a need for specialized conditioning to maintain the level of conditioning that the dancer has achieved. When performing, a dancer should engage in a daily technique class. The technique class should be particularly concered with a balance of strength in all the major muscles of the body as well as flexibility and endurance activities.

IMMEDIATE INJURY CARE

Often it is asked how a person can return to physical activity so quickly following a serious ligamentous sprain or muscle strain. The answer to this question is many faceted. A highly conditioned body heals more quickly than a poorly conditioned one; however, a highly conditioned body also deconditions rapidly when adequate activity is withdrawn. Also the individual who is seriously involved in a physical endeavor is highly motivated to get well and thus responds well to the therapies administered. In addition to these two factors, the most important factor in the response of healing is the immediacy of proper care. The application of cold, pressure, and elevation and the proper amount of rest immediately following an injury may mean the difference between a few days and several weeks of recovery time.

FOLLOW-UP CARE

Effective follow-up care of an injury involves knowing when to apply various therapies such as heat or cold and when to employ exercise. Each injury has certain individual characteristics and must be treated according to its own peculiarities; however, general concepts can be applied. For example, it is desirable that an injured dancer engage in general physical activity without aggravating the healing injured part. The continuance of an exercise program encourages injury healing and decreases the possibility of severe scarring. This does not mean, however, that a dancer should use the injured part before it is ready. A unique therapeutic strategy can be applied for each person and each injury type.

SUPPORTIVE TECHNIQUES

In the last ten years, the use of supportive techniques applied to physically active individuals has greatly increased. Strapping, special wraps, and padding can assist tremendously in the protection and healing process of many injuries if they are applied properly and at the appropriate time. Many strapping techniques protect a body part against additional injury and allow the dancer to engage more freely in general physical activity. Properly applied pads often can provide dancers with relief from pain and allow them to return to dancing faster than they could otherwise. It should be noted, however, that dance presents a unique problem in that a supportive or protective device should not detract from the impact of a performance by overly restricting motion or be so bulky as to be obvious to an audience.

Parts II, III, IV, and V of this book present a guide to the most effective application of the basic four for dance injuries.

II

WHY DANCE INJURIES?

Part II is devoted to the multifaceted problem of why dancers sustain injury in their chosen form of aesthetic endeavor. The three chapters presented in this section are designed to give the reader an overview of this question. These chapters include a discussion of the implications of body structure and composition, how the body is used, and the world that envelops and/or acts on the dancer.

3

Body structure and composition

The active person can sustain traumatic injuries by overstretching or abnormally compressing the body's tissues. These forces can result in injuries such as muscle strains, joint sprains, or even the more serious conditions of dislocations or fractures. Those qualities that allow the dancer's body to move freely and gracefully can also produce susceptibility to a variety of injuries. Although the human body has a great deal of structural strength, it also generally possesses many structural weaknesses that, when subjected to abnormal stress, can lead to injury. Besides the basic structure of the dancer's body, its total makeup or composition as determined by heredity and physical training also plays an important role.

MUSCLES

Muscles are those tissues within the body that are composed of bundles or sheets of fibers that contract and produce movement. Patterns of coordinated movement are dependent on the quality of muscle contraction and relaxation on the quality of pull on each bone where the muscle is attached and on the degree of stabilization by accessory or nonprime moving muscles at the stationary end of the one (Fig. 3-1). To function without injury in dance, muscles must have a high level of efficiency in the process of reciprocal inhibition, in which the muscles antagonistic to muscles that are moving the body are allowed to relax and stretch smoothly. If antagonist and agonist muscles receive simultaneous neural stimulation, movement cannot occur,

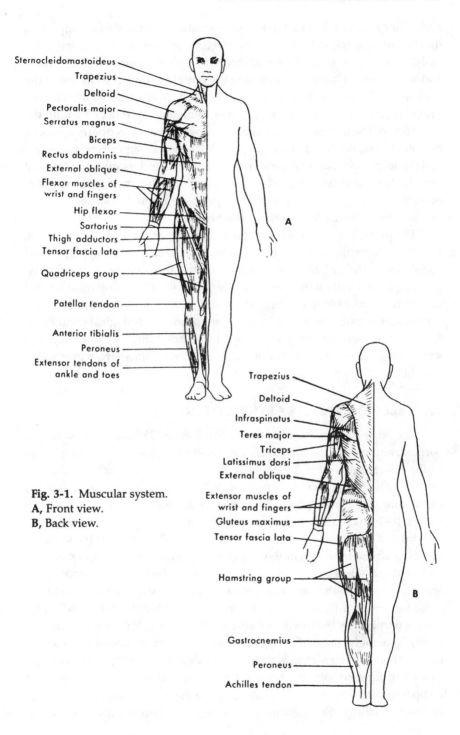

Sternocleidomastoideus
Trapezius
Deltoid
Pectoralis major
Serratus magnus
Biceps
Rectus abdominis
External oblique
Flexor muscles of wrist and fingers
Hip flexor
Sartorius
Thigh adductors
Tensor fascia lata
Quadriceps group
Patellar tendon
Anterior tibialis
Peroneus
Extensor tendons of ankle and toes

A

Trapezius
Deltoid
Infraspinatus
Teres major
Triceps
Latissimus dorsi
External oblique
Extensor muscles of wrist and fingers
Gluteus maximus
Tensor fascia lata
Hamstring group
Gastrocnemius
Peroneus
Achilles tendon

B

Fig. 3-1. Muscular system.
A, Front view.
B, Back view.

and injury may result. The stretch, or myotatic, reflex is also an important function of muscles, stabilizing and protecting joints as well as helping in the body's ability to balance. The stretch reflex occurs when a muscle is extended and subjected to a pull, at which time the muscle contracts to maintain the integrity of the joint with which it is associated. To ensure that muscles are providing maximum protection, patterns of movement must be within the capability of the individual dancer and strength must be properly balanced between those muscles that move a part and those that support related joints and guide the accuracy of the movement. It is well understood that physical exercise has a positive effect on cartilage, tendons, and ligaments, as well as on muscles. As a result, when exercise is properly applied it can help to serve as a protection to the body against injury.

The propelling force of the human body comes from its motor system, which includes the nerves and muscles. To be effective, muscles under conscious control of the brain must contract and release in synchrony, working reciprocally with their opposing muscles. Opposing muscles that do not relax effectively produce stress and abnormal tension in opposite muscles, eventually resulting in acute or chronic pathological conditions. Muscles also pad the body with their bulk, providing to the underlying structures protection against contusions or blows from sources external to the body.

THE SKELETON AND ITS ARTICULATIONS

The bony framework of the body consists of 206 individual bones. Of particular interest to the dancer are the bones of the feet and the long bones of the lower limbs (Fig. 3-2), which are susceptible to fractures. Also of interest is the particular structure of joints, which can facilitate or limit range of motion. In general, bones have relative strength based on two major factors: their shape and the changes of direction they may take. The strongest constructed long bone is one that is round and hollow, such as the femur in the thigh or the humerus in the upper arm. A bone that changes direction and/or shape—the clavicle, for example—is considered to have an anatomical weakness at that point and, in some cases, may be susceptible to fracture.

Like bones, articulations, or joints, have relative strengths and weaknesses, particularly the freely movable joints. Three factors provide articular strength; namely, skeletal design, ligamentous organization, and muscular organization. A deep socket, as opposed to a shallow socket, provides strength to a joint; for example, the hip joint has a very strong skeletal design as compared with the extremely weak design of the knee. Ligaments are bands or sheets of strong fibrous tissue that connect the articular ends of bones and

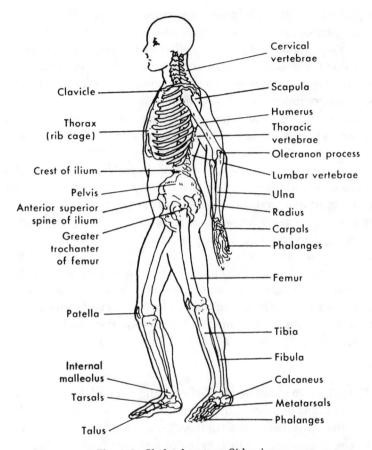

Clavicle

Thorax
(rib cage)

Crest of ilium

Pelvis

Anterior superior
spine of ilium

Greater
trochanter
of femur

Patella

Internal
malleolus

Tarsals

Talus

Cervical
vertebrae

Scapula

Humerus

Thoracic
vertebrae

Olecranon process

Lumbar vertebrae

Ulna

Radius

Carpals

Phalanges

Femur

Tibia

Fibula

Calcaneus

Metatarsals

Phalanges

Fig. 3-2. Skeletal system. Side view.

either enhance or limit movement. Ligaments are generally more dense in joint areas having the greatest stress. For example, greater stress is placed on the inner aspect of both the ankle and the knee; therefore, a much more dense and strong ligamentous arrangement appears on their outer aspects. Muscles can also provide joint strength when there is not a preponderance of long tendons crossing the joint, and the contractive tissue is closely associated with the joint. Therefore, from a muscular point of view the knee joint is a better example of a strong joint when compared with the ankle or wrist joint.

Feet

The articulations of the feet vary according to their location and particular function. In general, the foot is structured to bear weight and propel the body over terrain. To accomplish these ends, the foot is divided into three sections—forefoot, midfoot, and hindfoot—and is composed of 36 bones of different shapes and sizes joined together in 33 or more articulations. The forefoot is composed of 14 phalanges (toes) and five metatarsals. The toes are allowed hinge-type movement of flexion and extension, and the metatarsal bones are permitted some flexion and extension and slight movement from side to side as they joint the toes. The metatarsal articulations glide up and down as they join the midfoot, or tarsal, bones. The five tarsal bones composing the midfoot glide on each other. The two largest tarsal bones, the calcaneous (heel) and the talus, combine to make up the hindfoot. The calcaneus, which is the larger of the two, is designed to support weight and to provide a lifting or lowering of the inside of the foot (pronation/supination). These three foot regions are designed to form arches that give the foot flexibility, spring, and shock absorption and are presented as the inner, longitudinal, and transverse arches.

The strength of the foot is highly dependent on the maintenance of the interrelationship of muscle, muscle tendons, and ligaments. It is truly amazing that such a small and intricate mechanism as the foot is able to withstand the rigors of dance and, at the same time, is so important in determining the structural integrity of the entire body.

Ankles

The ankle is the joint that lies between the foot and the lower end of the leg. The fibula and tibia bones of the leg form a cuplike mortise over the talus, allowing the movements of flexion and extension but little, if any, lateral movement, depending on the degree of ligament laxity in the area. The ligaments that help to bind the ankle joint provide strong support on its medial (inner) aspect but much less support on is lateral (outer) aspect. In general, the weakest factor in the ankle joint is its musculature; with the exception of the calf muscle tendon or heel cord, the long tendons that cross all sides of the joint provide little strength. This anatomical weakness explains why ankle sprains are slow to rehabilitate and why, once disruption of supportive tissue has occurred, stability may have to be provided by outside elements such as special wraps or strappings.

Knees

The knee is designed to produce a hinge action. However, its skeletal makeup, in contrast to that of the ankle, is very weak; only a shallow recess is provided for each femoral condyle (articulating surface of the thigh bone) to rest on. Nature has assisted knee stability by providing two cartilaginous oval pieces that, like the discs between the vertebrae, assist in shock absorption and that also provide a slightly deeper socket for the femoral condyles. The knee, like the ankle, has its greatest ligamentous strength on its inner aspect (provided by the medial collateral ligaments), with a lighter and less dense ligamentous arrangement on the outer aspect. On the lateral aspect of the knee joint, the long fascial tendon of the faciae latae muscle gives additional support. It is paradoxical, however, that even with strong ligaments and musculature, injuries are more prevalent and usually more severe on the medial aspect of the knee. The knee is provided anterior-posterior (front-to-back) stabilization by the cruciate ligaments. By far the greatest strength of the knee joint, however, comes from its musculature. Muscles such as the quadriceps group, which extends the knee, the hamstring group, which flexes the knee, and the gastrocnemius muscles, which primarily point the toes and assist in bending the leg, all provide the knee joint with stability if conditioned properly.

When examining the knee joint, one must also consider the patella, a sesamoid bone that forms in the quadriceps extensor tendon. The patella protects the front of the knee and increases the leverage of the quadriceps muscle. Because it articulates only with the femur, a balance of pull on the patella by the quadriceps muscle is essential for smooth knee extension and flexion. A dancer who improperly performs a turn-out from the hip with the lower leg often distorts the muscle pull on the kneecap, causing it to misalign, and develops a pathological condition on the articular surface of the kneecap (see Chapter 5).

Hip

The hip joint is extremely important to the dancer. Anatomically it is one of the most stable joints in the body. A deep socket for the head of the femur provides a strong skeletal organization together with a heavy network of ligamentous and fibrous tissue that completely surrounds the hip joint (see Fig. 12-6). The support provided by this arrangement is increased by many strong intrinsic and extrinsic muscles. Basically the hip is extremely strong in all its anatomical features and is able to withstand a great many of the stresses placed on it by dance. It should be noted, however, that the hip is particularly vulnerable to injury in the flexed position. In flexion the hip joint loses stability and the articular capsule becomes lax, increasing its susceptibility to injury when placed in a stretch position, as when the dancer goes from passe to extension. It should also be noted that dance can place extreme stress on the normal integrity of the hip and its associated ligaments and muscles, resulting in pathomechanics and chronic injury.

Spine

The vertebral spine consists of many bones that, when combined, allow the trunk to move in many different directions. The areas of the spine most vulnerable to dance injury are the lumbosacral junction at the base of the vertebral column and the lumbar vertebrae located below the rib cage. At the lumbosacral junction, the movable spine makes contact with the very immobile pelvis. In general, the lumbar spine can be weak or strong, depending on the balance of musculature in the lower abdomen and lower back. The five lumbar vertebrae represent a strong skeletal and ligamentous structure, but like the lumbosacral junction, they are vulnerable to injury when weakness of the abdominal muscles is combined with tightness in the lower back region. Body mechanics plays an extremely important role in the prevention of lower back injuries and in determining whether the vertebral column and the pelvis are in good alignment.

The cervical region, or neck, does not have a very high incidence of injury in dance; however, occasionally a sudden twist or thrust will produce a muscle spasm and strain in this area. The cervical vertebrae are designed for full mobility. Consequently, they are not supported by a heavy bony design or ligamentous network. The greatest strength of the neck comes from its musculature. Therefore, if the muscles of the neck are not conditioned properly, they are prone to strain. Because the head, which commonly weighs from 9 to 12 pounds, may be moved suddenly and with great force in any direction, the neck musculature can be easily overstretched.

Upper limbs

Like the neck region, the shoulder girdle (which encompasses the articulations of the clavicle, the scapula and the head of the humerus, or shoulder joint) is designed for full mobility and not for support. The shoulder girdle gains its greatest strength from its musculature. Dance injuries of the shoulder girdle are primarily in the nature of sudden unrestrained muscle contractions and improper conditioning. Joints of the elbow, wrist, and hand do not have the same incidence of dance injury as other joints. However, they may be hurt by a fall on the outstretched arm. The elbow is a strong joint in every aspect with the exception of the radial joint, which allows movement of the forearm. The wrist derives its greatest strength from ligaments and muscle tendons.

In conclusion, the human body is mechanically designed for sustained and accurate movement. The upright posture of the human being provides the opportunity for the arms to work freely, since they are not necessary for support of the upper body as they are in the four-legged animal. The human body cannot be said to be designed for great feats of strength but for precision in fine and sensitive types of movement. Therefore, one must set forth the premise that when the dancer does not use the body according to its major design, injury is imminent. One may conclude that structurally the human body has relative strength in its skeleton, joints, and musculature and that humans vary in their structural strength depending on heredity, environment, and particular stresses imposed on their bodies.

4

Posture and body alignment

For the dancer, good body mechanics is essential to move efficiently and to defend against the possibility of injury (Fig. 4-1). Body mechanics is the functional relationship among the various body parts. For effective movement, each segment of the body must be in proper relationship to adjacent segments. With good posture, the body functions with the least amount of stress possible for each movement and for each body. Good body mechanics is relative to the type of activity being engaged in, such as sitting, standing, walking, and dancing, as well as to the type of body build that the individual is endowed with. Consequently, there is no normal posture that fits every individual. To maintain proper alignment, the human body must continually combat the force of gravity as it is being pulled toward the center of the earth. Body segments that are misaligned react to gravity more adversely than segments that are in good alignment. In essence, proper body mechanics reflects good balance and a small amuont of strain on the supporting and moving structures.

The center of gravity of the human body is also an essential factor in good postural alignment. This center is usually found at a point in the middle of the pelvis, approximately dividing the individual in half. Men normally have longer legs and a higher center of gravity, whereas women normally have shorter lower limbs and a lower center of gravity.

STABILITY VS. INSTABILITY

Standing upright on two feet provides a very small base of support;

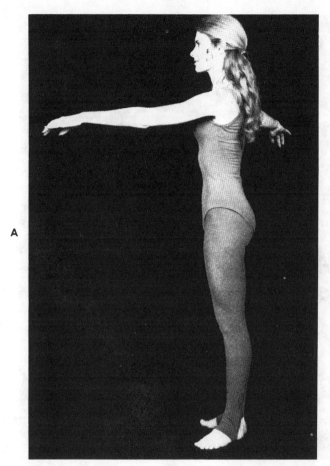

Fig. 4-1. A,Good body mechanics is essential for efficient movement and defense against injury.

consequently, the body is relatively unstable in its normal standing position. Whether standing in one position or moving, the body is always striving to offset the pull of gravity. It is obvious, therefore, that the most stable position of the body is when it is aligned over its own base of support. The closer the body's center of gravity is to the center of its base of support, the better the equilibrium. Body movement is often the purposeful gaining and losing of the base of support. "In the human animal, the walk is the key pattern of fall and recovery, . . . that is, the giving in to and rebounding from gravity. This is the very core of all movement, in my opinion. The human body constantly fluctuates between the resistance to and yielding to gravity."[12]

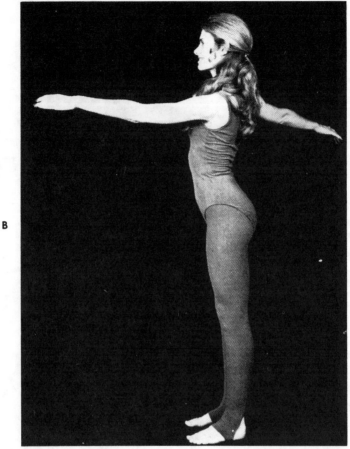

B

Fig. 4-1, cont'd. B, Faulty body mechanics results in inefficient movement and a susceptibility to injury.

In addition to the reciprocal relationship of ligaments and muscles, many other factors within the human organism are designed to maintain postural alignment. For example, postural positioning in dynamic movement is controlled by visual cues in terms of the body's position in space. The semicircular canals in the inner ear provide information on the body's position to the brain. There are also receptors in the tendons, joints, and muscles that provide continual information to the brain and proprioceptors as to the body's relative position in space. Any malfunction of these organs individually or in relationship to one another can result in temporary or chronic problems that can cause serious postural malalignments and loss of movement efficiency, followed by an increased susceptibility to injury and eventual chronic orthopedic problems in later life. To the dancer, good postural alignment is essential for career longevity and freedom from acute and chronic handicapping injuries.

GOOD STANDING POSTURE

As described, good posture in an efficient body and motor system allows for the maximum functioning of the body with expenditure of the least energy. Although the body is seldom in a static position, posture is often discussed in this way to provide examples of good alignment (Fig. 4-2). In the standing position the body weight is equally spread over the feet, with equal pressure placed on the various parts of the foot such as the heel and the ball of

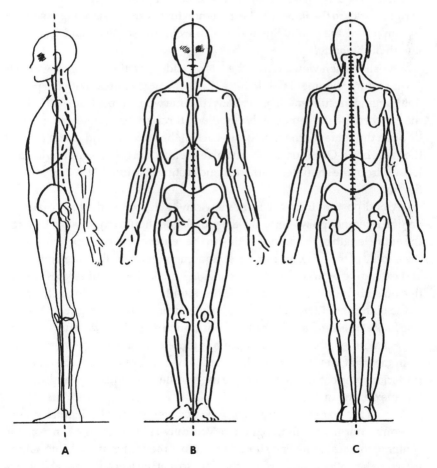

A   B   C

Fig. 4-2. Normal postural alignment. **A,** Side view. **B,** Front view. **C,** Back view.

the foot. The five toes provide some assistance in the equalization of pressure. Balanced equally over the feet are the lower legs, which sit comfortably on top of the axis of each ankle, called the talus. Although the legs are straight, the knees are not maintained in a stiff or locked position. On top of the legs is the pelvis, balanced in such a manner that the muscles of the abdomen, lower back, and thighs are in equal contraction. The pelvis, in coordination with the lumbar spine, allows for a normal amount of anterior-posterior curvature. The upper back, supported primarily by the thoracic vertebrae, also has the proper amount of anterior-posterior curvature to be balanced with the lower lumbar spine. Resting comfortably on the thorax is the shoulder girdle, with the arms hanging in a straight line down the sides of the trunk. Sitting on top of the cervical spine, the head is positioned in such a manner that its weight is distributed equally in front and in back. In such a balanced position the jaw is at right angles to the floor. The best method to determine standing posture is by employing the plumb line test, with a weighted string extending the full length of the body.

Ideally, when viewed from the lateral (side) position, a person who has good posture alignment would have the following features. With the plumb line hanging the full length of the body, the line would cross from just behind the ear, through the center of the shoulder, through the middle of the pelvis, through the center of the hip, just in back of the kneecap, and just in front of the ankle bone. One must also scrutinize the arm hang. The arm should hang loosely from the shoulder, with the hand resting comfortably at the center of the hip.

Good posture from the front view can be determined by a horizontal-vertical reference point. Vertically the plumb line should cross evenly through the entire length of the body, starting in the center of the head, passing down the middle of the nose, mouth, chest, abdomen (or linea alba), the umbilicus, and extending between the two legs. Horizontally the shoulder tips should line up with one another; the nipple line should be even; the top of the hips, or the ilium, should be in line; and the kneecaps should be aligned. One can also look at the arm hang in the front position to determine whether the arms are equal in length. It is also important to determine leg alignment across from the front view. To do so, the plumb line is dropped from the anterior-posterior spine of the ilium, crossing the middle of the kneecaps and striking the apex of the instep.

From the rear view one also must look at vertical and horizontal lines to determine normal postural alignment. Vertically a plumb line is taken from the center of the head. The line should then cross the center of the spine, falling between the buttocks and striking the floor so that the feet are of equal distance from the plumb line. The back view can also indicate to the observer whether the shoulders are level and if the scapulae are in horizontal alignment.

Of extreme importance to the entire body is the proper alignment of the foot, ankle, and leg (Figs. 4-3 and 4-4). Like the other segmental relationships of the body, the foot and ankle must be properly aligned if the complicated system of tendons and muscles is to work efficiently. Because the foot is the base of support for the entire body, faulty alignment here can cause postural deviations in the other mechanical systems of the body. An ideal relationship of the bony segments of the foot and leg produces the maximum efficiency during standing and locomotion. In the standing posture the lower third of

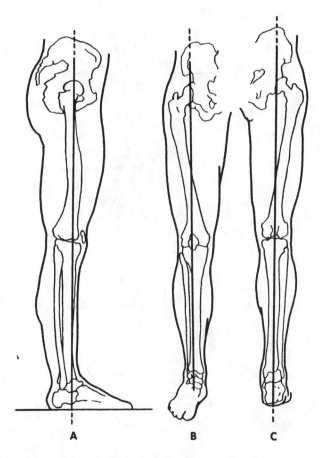

A   **B**   **C**

Fig. 4-3. Normal leg and foot alignment. **A,** Side view. **B,** Front view. **C,** Back view.

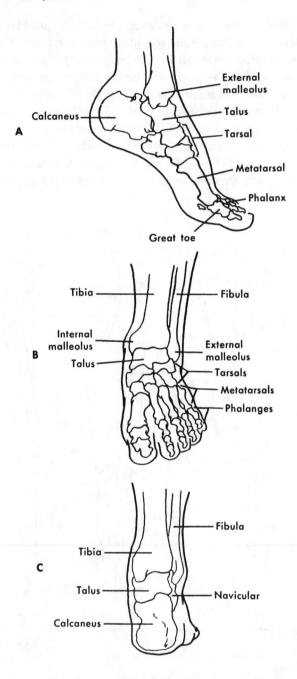

Fig. 4-4. Proper bony relationships of the foot. **A,** Side view. **B,** Front view. **C,** Back view.

the leg rests on the talus, which in turn rests directly on the heel bone, or calcaneus. The talus and the calcaneus represent the hindfoot, or tarsus. The midfoot, or lesser talus, which in turn rests directly on the heel bone, or calcaneus, consists of the navicular, cuboid, and three cuniform bones; the five metatarsals and the five phalanges constitute the forefoot. In movement in the upright position, weight is transferred forward on the foot to the three cuniform bones and the cuboid and then to the metatarsals and phalanges. In the normal standing position the body weight is carried on the heel and the forefoot, with weight being distributed equally throughout the heads of the five metatarsal bones. The toes also assist in balancing the body as their bottom surfaces come in full contact with the floor.

The foot also has several arches that provide for normal functioning and protection. Longitudinal arches are found on the medial and lateral aspects of the foot. The inside, or medial, longitudinal arch extends from the anterior aspect of the heel to the distal heads of the metatarsal bones, whereas the normally smaller lateral longitudinal arch extends from the heel to the distal head of the fifth metatarsal. An extremely important arch in the forepart of the foot is the metatarsal arch, which is dome shaped and formed by the front heads of the metatarsal bones. In general, a healthy foot is one that is well articulated and flexible and has strong ligaments and good muscle tone. For the dancer, the normally aligned foot is one of the most important physical assets.

EXAMINING POSTURE

All persons concerned with dance should have an understanding of basic screening methods in determining body alignment and misalignment. The most common techniques utilized for screening postural alignment are the grid, the plumb line, and various special devices to determine leg, ankle, and foot alignment.

The posture grid may be composed of a network of 2-inch squares or, as seen in Fig. 4-5, 6-inch rectangles suspended on an angular frame 7½ feet long and 3 feet wide. Dividing the grid into equal halves at the center is a line, usually of a different color or width. This center line is equivalent to the plumb line. The vertical or horizontal lines of the posture screen provide various reference points. In determining body segment alignment or misalignment, the inspector can observe the dancer either as a total entity or in segments.

In using the posture screen, the inspector should have the dancer wear as little clothing as possible. The typical dance costume of leotards and tights is permissable for scanning the general contours of the body, but when it

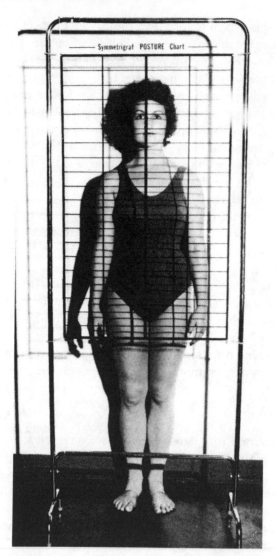

Fig. 4-5. Determining postural deviations through the use of a grid.

comes to observing the back, shoulders, and legs, it is desirable to have the bony landmarks revealed. The dancer is screened from three views: the side, back, and front. For the observation the dancer takes a position approximately 12 inches behind the screen and stands so that the center line of the grid crosses the midline of the body. The dancer's feet are then positioned with the heels approximately 2 inches apart and the feet slightly abducted (turned out). In the side view position the dancer stands so that the center line of the screen strikes just in front of the lateral malleolus (ankle bone). In the back view position the dancer stands with the back to the screen approximately 12 inches from the screen, with the heels 2 inches apart and feet slightly turned out. The dancer is instructed to stand as naturally as possible while being viewed.

Postural deviations that are determined by reading the grid are normally indicated in terms of mild, moderate, or severe or in degrees of deviation. When the body is viewed as a whole, 1 degree is equivalent to 1 inch, 2 degrees to 2 inches, and 3 degrees to 3 inches of deviation. When one part of the body is observed as it relates to another, ½ inch, 1 inch, 1½ inches refer to 1, 2, and 3 degrees of deviation, respectively. These areas are the chest and the region of the ankle and foot. Many other body areas must be scrutinized subjectively rather than by use of the posture screen as a definitive examining device (Table 1).

Table 1. Posture screen and degree of deviation

Condition	Degree of severity
Front view	
Side body lean	1 inch = 1 degree
Head tilt	½ inch = 1 degree
Shoulder height	½ inch = 1 degree
Linea alba	½ inch = 1 degree
Side pelvic tilt	½ inch = 1 degree
Knock-knees (legs together, distant ankles apart)	½ inch = 1 degree
Tibial torsion (kneecap deviates from center line)	½ inch = 1 degree
Side view	
Front or back body lean	1 inch = 1 degree
Forward or backward head	½ inch = 1 degree
Forward or backward shoulders	½ inch = 1 degree
Round back (kyphosis)	½ inch = 1 degree
Lordosis, flat back, forward or backward pelvis	½ inch = 1 degree
Bent or back knee	½ inch = 1 degree
Back view	
Scoliosis (cervical, thoracic, and lumbar)	½ inch = 1 degree
Bowlegs (legs together, distant knees apart)	½ inch = 1 degree

The inspector normally stands approximately 12 feet from the dancer, who is behind the screen. From this distance the entire body can be seen. While the dancer takes each of the three prescribed positions, the inspector first looks at the entire body for leaning and whole body distortion and then views the body segmentally either from foot to head or vice versa.

The relationships are of the head to the shoulder, the trunk to the pelvis, the pelvis to the thigh, and the thigh to the lower leg. The posture grid method for determining postural anomalies gives only one indication of gross or obvious inadequacies and should not be used as a definitive diagnostic tool. The static standing position assumed behind the screen is not a usual human attitude; therefore, extreme caution should be taken by the observer when definitive statements are made as to the seriousness of specific postural divergencies. The plumb line is an excellent tool in determining lateral deviations, front midline deviations, and back midline deviations. It is also valuable in determining vertical leg alignment.

FOOT EXAMINATION

The foot examination is more difficult than screening other segments of the body. However, two tests can be used by the layperson to determine proper alignment of the foot and ankle. These tests, although not equivalent to examination by a physician, can indicate to the observer conditions that may need further examination. The first of the instruments used is the pedograph (Fig. 4-6). The pedograph print is similar to a fingerprint except that it is of the foot under weight-bearing conditions. The subject is instructed to walk up to the pedograph and step on it in a normal manner. The pedograph in turn makes an ink impression of the foot on a paper recording form. Although not a definitive screening device that would normally be used in medicine, this device does reveal weight-bearing characteristics and indicates the position of the toes, the relative height of the longitudinal arch, and the relative position of the metatarsal arch.

Another excellent tool is the podiascope (Fig. 4-7), a boxlike device made of wood with a ½-inch glass top and a reflecting mirror inside. The subject stands on the glass top while pressure from the weight bearing is reflected in the mirror for observation by the examiner. Weight-bearing areas are reflected as pale white areas. Besides weight bearing, the examiner can also observe a number of other foot features; namely, the general position of the longitudinal and the metatarsal arches and the relationship of the Achilles tendon to the calcaneus. The observer can also readily see if there is abnormal callus formation on the foot.

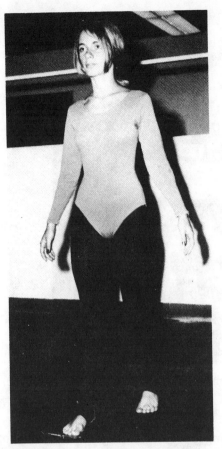

Fig. 4-6. Taking a foot impression on the pedograph.

Walking examination. Besides the stationary examination procedures mentioned, walking analysis provides a dynamic means of determining postural integrity of the body. Foot and leg functions are particularly visible in the walking action. Observing shoe wear is also an excellent means of determining how the dancer bears weight during walking. An older shoe will normally display wear on the outside of the heel and on the big toe side of the ball joint. To make a general determination of walking form, observe the dancer from the back as he or she walks away from 15 or 20 paces and from the back as he or she returns to the starting position. This procedure should be repeated until all the desired alignment factors have been observed. However, more attention should be paid to the function of leg swings and foot positions. The following factors should be observed:

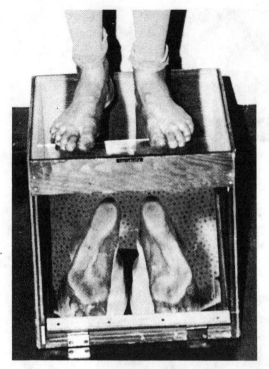

Fig. 4-7. Weight-bearing characteristics indicated by the podiascope.

1. Legs should swing forward in a straight pattern with both kneecaps centered between the femur and the lower leg.
2. The distance between the feet should allow for a fluid forward movement without excess motion of the hips, either sideways or in rotation.
3. The position of each foot is either straight or slightly abducted when contact is made with the surface.
4. Initial contact is made on the back outside of the heel, which is responsible for the wearing down of the outside of the shoe.
5. The weight on the foot then shifts from the heel and outer side of the sole to the metatarsal joint (ball joint), with the big toe side predominating.
6. Pushing off for the next step may now involve the entire ball joint equally, or the fifth metatarsal may be accentuated.

The walking examination is especially valuable when one is observing a dancer with pronated feet, tibial torsion, and/or knock-knees.

Foot squeeze test. Ideally, a healthy foot, free of structural problems, will feel soft and pliable, somewhat like a young child's foot when the forefront is squeezed (Fig. 4-8). As weight-bearing problems creep into the dancer's habits, the foot becomes increasingly rigid when squeezed. In application of the foot squeeze test, the following subjective indicators can be used: a forefoot that has some resistance to being squeezed but still feels pliable and soft to the touch may be considered as first degree; a forefoot that feels tight and somewhat unyielding to squeezing is considered as a second degree; and one that feels extremely hard and tight and almost completely resists being squeezed is considered as third degree. In general, the first-degree deviation must be considered a functional problem that can be aided with exercise and proper reeducation. Second-degree deviation, on the other hand, is in the transitional stage where exercise and re-education may be of some benefit, but full recovery should not be expected. In third-degree forefoot, in many instances it is doubtful whether remediation will be of much value.

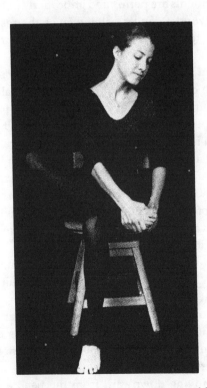

Fig. 4-8. The squeeze test determines the degree of forefoot rigidity.

POSTURAL PROBLEMS IN DANCE

From birth to death the human organism is resisting the force of gravity. The newborn baby lying in the crib is almost completely overcome by the pressure of gravity and unable to do anything but remain in a recumbent position. As the musculature and skeletal system mature, the infant is eventually able to overcome gravity and assume an upright posture. Gravity is continually forcing the individual toward the center of the earth. The ultimate upright posture demands specific strength of major antigravity muscles such as the erector muscles of the spine (erector spinae), the quadriceps group, and the gastrocnemius. Ideally the mature person resists gravity through symmetrical and synchronous muscular development. When improper use of the body is undertaken before the physiological readiness exists to withstand the rigors of a particular stressful activity—which sometimes happens in ballet—the body will assume faulty habits.

Dance, like any strenuous, repetitious activity, can provide the performer with an outstanding opportunity to develop a well-conditioned body. On the other hand, if dance movements are performed improperly or if movements are attempted that are beyond a dancer's ability level, the result may be a breakdown of supporting structures followed by serious postural deviations or injury.

Forward head/cervical lordosis. Many postural deviations are obvious from the side view. These deviations are more technically called anterior-posterior deviations. The first and probably most common is forward head. In this situation the ear appears in front of the plumb line rather than in good alignment. The individual in this abnormal position develops weakness in the extensor cervical muscles that keep the head erect and develops a shortening of the flexor muscles in the front of the neck. Occasionally the forward head becomes incorrectly realigned by development of cervical lordosis, or accentuation of the normal curve of the neck (Fig. 4-9). In this situation the dancer would appear to have normal alignment except that the chin would jut upward instead of being parallel to the floor.

In correcting forward head, the dancer must strengthen the extensor muscles of the neck, stretch the flexors, and learn to maintain the proper position. It is suggested that the dancer try to push the head upward as if a rod were holding the head on top of the shoulders. Correction of cervical lordosis can be attained by much the same procedure; however, the dancer must attempt to decrease the curve of the neck by performing various neck and back flattening exercises (see Fig. 6-8).

Forward shoulders. Moving downward from the head and neck, the examiner next scans the thorax and shoulder complex. The common deviation in this area is forward shoulders, in which the shoulders are forward of

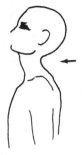

Fig. 4-9. Cervical lordosis.

the plumb line. In this situation muscular tightness exists in the chest region and a stretching and weakening of the muscles in the upper back region. Often associated with forward shoulders are winged scapulae, caused by the scapulae being pulled outward from the rib cage.

Round back; kyphosis. A more serious condition in the upper trunk region, often associated with forward shoulders, is an exaggerated spinal curve called round back or kyphosis (Fig. 4-10). Kyphosis of the thoracic spine is an abnormal rounding of the upper back that produces much the same type of muscular imbalance seen in forward shoulders: tight musculature in the chest that overpowers the weaker muscles of the upper back, particularly the erector spinae muscles, which maintain the spine in an erect position. Overcoming these conditions of the upper trunk requires a stretching and lengthening of the musculature in the chest region and a strengthening of the erector spinae muscles and the posterior aspect of the shoulder girdle (see Fig. 6-28).

Swayback; lumbar lordosis. Lumbar lordosis is a common postural deviation of the lumbar spine and pelvis in which the normal forward curve of the lumbar spine is accentuated (Fig. 4-11). This condition often results in a forward tilting of the pelvis, adding to the swaybacked appearance that is characteristic of many dancers. Because this area is very near the center of gravity, many muscles are involved. Normally the pelvis is maintained in its balance position by an even pull of the abdominal, lumbosacral, and hip flexor muscles together with the muscles of the thigh and hip. However, in lumbar lordosis the abdominal muscles are weaker than the muscles of the lumbar spine, which are usually contracted and tight, and the hamstring muscles. Also, in lordosis the rectus femoris muscles of the quadriceps group usually are tight along with the iliopsoas muscle. This muscular inbalance results in the pulling down of the pelvis anteriorly, creating the typical swayback or forward pelvic tilt. The dancer with this problem will find difficulty in lifting the leg such as the grande battement (leg kick) or a develope (leg extension). Performance of the plie also is adversely affected.[16]

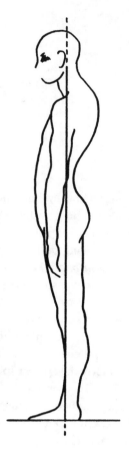

Fig. 4-10. Kyphosis of the thoracic spine.

Overcoming lordosis requires a great deal of hard work involving stretching the lower back, the hip flexors, and the hamstring muscles and strengthening the abdominal muscles in a concerted effort to re-establish lumbar, pelvic, and leg alignment (see Fig. 6-27). Because the iliopsoas muscle is so closely related to the lordotic curve of the lumbar vertebrae, stretching this muscle alone often realigns this area dramatically (see Fig. 6-5).

Forward or backward pelvic tilt. The pelvis is closely associated with the relative position of the lumbar spine. A straight line can be drawn between the anterior-posterior and posterior-superior spine of the ilium. If the pelvis is inclined forward, it is said to be a forward pelvic tilt, and if inclined backward, a posterior tilt. The same muscles that are closely associated with lumbar lordosis also affect the tipping either forward or backward of the pelvis.

Flat back. Flat back often is a condition opposite to lordosis in terms of specific muscle imbalance. It results in a flattening of the lower back and a

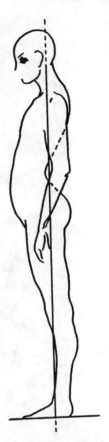

Fig. 4-11. Lumbar lordosis.

posterior (backward) tilt of the pelvis and/or elongation of the thoracic curve (Fig. 4-12). Correction of flat back involves strengthening of the lower back and hip flexors and stretching the abdominal and hamstring muscles.

Leg problem. Closely associated with the relative position of the pelvis and vertebral column are the thigh and lower legs. As described earlier, in a normal lateral alignment of the legs the plumb line falls from the center of the hip, crossing just behind the patella and just in front of the outer malleolus. A plumb line that falls in front of the patella may reveal a condition called back knees, or genu recurvatum (Fig. 4-13). This problem is very closely associated with lordosis and the forward tilt of the pelvis frequently found in ballet dancers. Back knee is produced by an imbalance in the strength of the quadriceps, hamstring, and gastrocnemius muslces. The gastrocnemius and quadriceps overpower the hamstrings, pulling the leg and thigh back into a hyperextended position. To overcome back knee a great deal of effort must

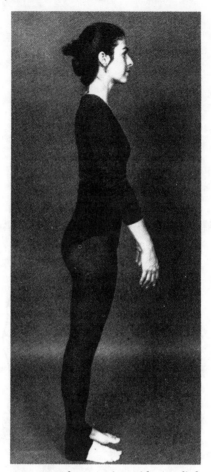

Fig. 4-12. Some dancers may produce a spine with very little curves that is sometimes called a flat back.

be expended to realign the hip, thigh, and lower leg, with special attention given to strengthening the hamstrings.

On the other hand, if the plumb line falls well behind the patella, the knee is in a hyperflexed position, indicating tight and constricted hamstring muscles (see Fig. 4-13, B). In contrast to the treatment of back knee, the hamstrings of the hyperflexed knee should be stretched and lengthened to restore the proper alignment. The hyperflexed knee may be characteristics of the individual with flat back.

The student of posture must be aware that a deviation in any one segment of the body can produce additional deviations in many other parts of the body. For example, a dancer with chronic forward head could, as a

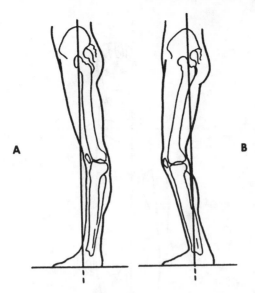

Fig. 4-13. Side view of leg malalignments. **A,** Back knees. **B,** Hyperflexed knees.

result, develop forward shoulders, kyphosis, lordosis, and hyperextended knees.

Tilting seen on front view. In viewing the body from the front, the observer should study both the vertical and horizontal components. Scanning the body in its entirety should determine if there is a left or right tilt. Body tilting may be the result of faulty habits or of a shortened leg (Fig. 4-14).

Studying the segments of the body from head to foot, the observer may find many deviations common in dancers. In relationship to the shoulders, the head may be tilted left or right or it may be twisted. Head tilt, as with whole body tilt, demands a reeducation of the proper sense of positioning. In the more severe cases, reeducation must be combined with a proper exercise program that includes stretching of the contracted side and strengthening of the elongated side of the neck. Viewing the body from the front can reveal many aberrations of the shoulders, shoulder girdle, and arms. For example, one shoulder can be higher than the other or both shoulders can be abnormally high because of contracted musculature on both sides of the upper shoulder region. Shoulders that are uneven or asymmetrical can result from a curvature in the spine or can occur because of some abnormality within the shoulder complex. If the origin of deviation is within the shoulder musculature, it is important that the contracted side be stretched and the lower side be strengthened along with reeducation exercises. Specific distortions of the trunk can be discerned by such signs as an uneven nipple line or an off-center linea alba

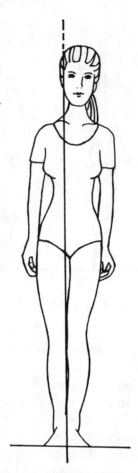

Fig. 4-14. Sideward body tilt.

(center line created by the coming together of the abdominal muscles). An uneven hang of the arms may indicate an abnormal deviation of the thorax and vertebral column.

Lateral pelvic tilt. Lateral pelvic tilt, a condition in which the pelvis is low on one side and high on the other, can be detected from both the front and back views. This condition is usually associated with contracted muscles in the lower back attributed to uneven leg length. Kneecaps that are not level often reveal a shortening of one leg. This type of asymmetry should be routinely referred to a physician for more accurate assessment and remediation. Front view screening is best for determining leg alignment, because key landmarks such as the anterior-superior spine of the ilium, the kneecap, and the foot are more easily discerned from the front.

Leg deviation. Three leg deviations are common among dancers. These are tibial torsion (a twisting of the lower leg bones), bowlegs, or genu varus (Fig. 4-15). Tibial torsion is best determined by examining the position of the kneecap. In most cases the kneecap of the dancer with tibial torsion is rotated inward with the foot pointing straight ahead. Less often the foot is pointed straight ahead while the kneecap is rotated outward. Because this is a condition involving the entire leg, correction involves the ankle, knee, and hip. Commonly the outward rotators of the hip and thigh are weak in comparison to the inward rotators, which are tight and need to be stretched. Dancers with this problem should be identified early and referred to a specialist for shoe correction and remedial exercises. This condition can be caused by the young dancer performing pliés incorrectly with the knee turned inward and the foot outward. Another major cause of tibial torsion is when the dancer consistently performs a turn-out incorrectly. Rather than properly turning out from the hip, the dancer completes the movement by rotating the lower leg outward.

Both knock-knees and bowlegs are determined in terms of how the legs are aligned. The knock-kneed dancer displays the ability to touch the medial

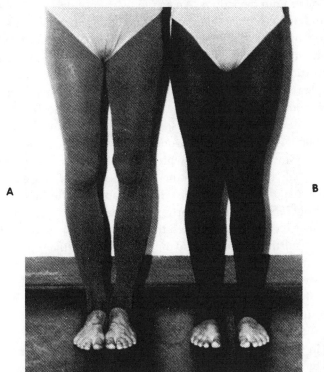

Fig. 4-15. Leg deviations. **A,** Bowlegs (genu varum). **B,** Knock-knees (genu valgum).

femoral condyles (insides of the knees) but is unable to touch the insides of the ankle bones. In this situation the lower legs are abducted (turned out from the midline of the body). On the other hand, the dancer who has bowlegs is unable to touch the insides of the knees while touching together the insides of the ankles. This produces a bowed appearance in the legs.

Correction of leg alignment problems is very difficult and requires the advice of a physician. In the early stages of the problem, corrective shoe devices that help tight musculature to be extended and weak musculature to become strengthened are usually the treatments of choice. The dancer must make sure that exercises or dance patterns engaged in do not accentuate the leg alignment problem.

Often associated with bowlegs are high longitudinal arches, supinated ankles with feet inverted, hyperextended knees and an inward rotation of the thighs. Conversely, with knock-knees the longitudinal arches are low, the ankles are often pronated with the feet everted, and there is an outward rotation of the thighs. In both bowlegs and knock-knees, correction should include proper footwear and must be conducted early in life if remediation is to occur. Dancers who abnormally stress their bodies very early in life often develop lower limb deviations. An astute teacher of dance will make sure that all students are physically mature enough to withstand the physical rigors paced on them by particular techniques. It is of the utmost importance that an attempted dance skill not be deliterious to a maturing dancer's normal postural development.

Winged scapula and scoliosis. The most postural anomalies that can be discerned from the back are winged scapula and scoliosis. The winged scapula is a deviation that displays an abduction or pulling away of the shoulder blade from the thorax, producing a wing effect. This problem is very common among thin dancers with a generally weak shoulder girlde and is often naturally overcome when the individual begins to use the arms in hanging and support activities. The winged scapula is often associated with forward shoulders caused by overly strong pectoral muscles and can be remedied by exercises that lengthen the chest muscles and strengthen the muscles that pull the scapula toward the spinal column (the rhomboid major muscles).

Scoliosis is the most serious of all postural deviations. It is a lateral deviation of the spinal column that causes an asymmetry of the thorax, pelvis, and upper and lower limbs. Curvature of the spine can be detected from the back view and appears as a "C" or "S" curve (Fig. 4-16). As was indicated in the discussion of the front view deviations, asymmetry that is produced by a scoliotic curve is often reflected in the frontview by an uneven nipple line, uneven arm hand, and a linea alba that deviates left or right from

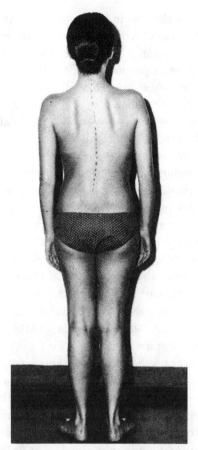

Fig. 4-16. "S"-curve scoliosis.

the center posture screen line. There may also appear to be a laterial hip tilt. A "C" curve is commonly called a simple curve, and as all curves are indicated as to direction, it is named for its convex side. A "C" curve that has attempted to compensate for the deviation is comonly called an "S" curve. However, the "S" compensation is usually incomplete, leaving the dancer with a great deal of asymmetry throughout the body. Because the causes of lateral spinal deviation are numerous, varied, and often unknown, it is usually not detected until the individual is in late childhood or early adolescence, often too late to make permanent corrections. In many cases the dance teacher will be the one to detect this type of problem and should immediately refer the student to a physician. In the early stages of scoliosis the primary problem is functional, involving only one soft tissue, and can often be corrected by proper treatment. As the condition progresses, the problem becomes a combination of soft-tissue and permanent skeletal and ligamentous changes that are difficult if not impossible to completely correct. Dance can be an outstanding means of ameliorating scoliosis, because it demands an ability for symmetry of movement. Unilateral activities, particularly those that exert a strong pull on the side of the curve, should be avoided at all costs.

Several tests can be initiated by the screener to determine whether scoliosis is present. The first is to very carefully palpate and mark with a grease pencil each spinous process of the dancer. Observation of this line may reveal the presence of a curvature. If so, the dancer should bend forward from the waist, allowing the arms to hang down. Two factors are observed while the dancer is in this position: (1) whether the spine straightens out in this position and (2) whether the thorax appears to be elevated more on one side than the other. If the spine straightens out while the dancer is bent over, it may indicate that the problem is functional, or involving primarily soft muscle tissue. If the curve only partly straightens out, then the condition may be considered transitional, or consisting of a combination of pliable soft tissue and permanently curved bone structures. If there is no straightening, the problem may be completely fixated in deformed bone. If the rib cage is higher on one side, it may indicate a twisting of the thorax as a result of the lateral deviation of the spine (Fig. 4-17).

It is advisable to check the dancer's leg length when scoliosis is suspected or has been determined by examination. Uneven length of the long bones of the legs is a major indicator of scoliosis in late childhood and early adolescence. Although definitive determination of uneven leg length must come from a physician, the dance instructor can make a subjective observation of the problem and subsequently refer the dancer to the proper professional source. The test is given with the dancer lying in a supine position with legs together and arms at the sides. The examiner stands at the dancer's feet and grasps the dancer's ankles with palms resting just under the medical malleolus of each ankle. After pulling gently to completely lengthen the legs the examiner determines whether the medial ankle bones are lined up. While both legs are being observed, the examiner also makes a determination of whether the patella and the anterior spine of the ilium of each leg appear to be even.

Persons usually develop some asymmetry in their bodies because of hand dominance and the use of one side of the body in preference to the other. Therefore, the majority of persons might be said to have some minor postural deviations contributing to scoliosis. However, to the dancer even the most minute asymmetry may eventually result in a serious acute injury or perhaps permanent chronic physical limitations and eventual elimination from the dance profession.

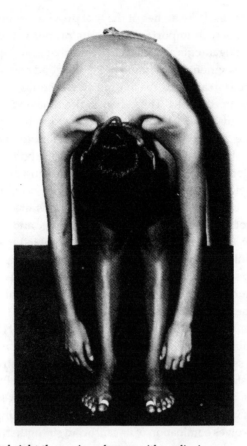

Fig. 4-17. Elevated right thorax in a dancer with scoliosis.

FOOT MALALIGNMENT AND STRUCTURAL PROBLEMS

The feet and legs are the primary tools of dance and must function at their optimum level in order for them to be highly responsive to the will of the dancer. The feet are mentioned last in this chapter but are not considered least in importance, because foot problems can be a detriment to the efficient functioning of the entire body. Painful feet can be devastating to the dancer's career. Consequently, it is necessary that problems of the feet, particularly mechanical defects, be overcome as soon as possible before permanent impairment occurs. Such factors as good hygiene, maintaining muscles in proper condition, and properly fitting shoes and socks are of the utmost importance to those who desire to maintain their feet in top health.

Arches. In general, the arches of the foot provide proper positioning of various foot bones with important segments properly aligned to prevent overstretching of ligaments and ensure the normal functioning of muscles. The primary foot segments that should be kept in good position are the seven irregularly shaped tarsal bones, the five metatarsal bones, and the 14 phalanx bones that make up the toes. These bones, the tibia and fibula (lower leg bones), and the talus bone of the ankle must be properly aligned in the static standing posture as well as in the dynamic locomotor postures. Arches provide a shock-absorbing protection to the rest of the body and also provide a space for tendons and other structures without being overly impinged as the result of weight bearing. Ideally the dancer is seeking an extremely strong and flexible foot, which implies that bones are properly placed, ligaments are not abnormally stretched, and intrinsic and extrinsic muscles are in good tone. Contrary to what has been thought in the past, arches that have begun to fall are very difficult to restore to proper height with exercise. Therefore, early signs of foot problems must be acted on before permanent structural deviations have taken place. Concern for the maintenance of arch integrity must be given when pain first arises.

Flatfeet. Pes planus (flatfoot) refers to the lowering of the border of the medial longitudinal arch (Fig. 4-18). It occurs when, because of improper afoot attire, excess weight, or improper use of the foot, the structures that had once provided stabilization allow the medial longitudinal arch to fall. The problem is often associated with the pronated foot, knock-knees, and tibial torsion. Persons having this problem may toe-out in walking. Amelioration of pes planus involves elimination of its cause and strengthening of weakened muscles. Exercise that encourages a curling downward action of toes may help prevent further drooping of the arch (see Figs. 6-17 and 6-18). With the falling of the longitudinal arch and the tendency of the foot to pronate, muscles on the lateral aspect of the foot, the peroneal group, tend to shorten

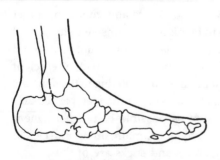

Fig. 4-18. Pes planus (flatfoot).

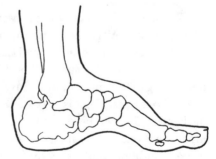

Fig. 4-19. Pes cavus (high arch).

along with the gastrocnemius and soleus muscles, which help to point the foot. The dancer with longitudinal arch problems should be discouraged from dancing on hard, rigid surfaces for long periods and encouraged to do activities on soft, resilient kinds of material such as grass or sand.

High arch. The opposite of pes planus is the problem of pes cavus (Fig. 4-19), or very high longitudinal arch. In this condition, abnormal stress is placed on the instep, ball of the foot, and heel. Pes cavus is usually assocaited with heavy callus formation on the plantar aspect of the heel and the ball of the foot as a result of the increased stresses in these areas. If pain is associated with this problem, referral should be made to a foot specialist.

The pronated foot. The pronated foot is often associated with ankle deviation; however, it is primarily within the forefoot and is a dual problem of foot abduction and eversion. In this problem there is a strain on the medial border of the longitudinal arch. This deviation also results in a faulty relationship of the talus, calcaneus and talus, and phalangeal articulations. Inspection from the rear of the pronated ankle often reveals a bowing medial-ward of the Achilles tendon. This condition is called Helbing's sign (Fig. 4-20). Prolonged condition of the foot frequently produces other deviations such as knock-knees and deviations in the hip region. The opposite of the pronated foot is the supinated foot, which is often associated with bowlegs and pes cavus. Remediation of pronated feet involves realignment of the knee and specific exercises to strengthen the arch.

Metatarsal and toe problems. Other problems common to the foot are painful conditions that center about the metatarsal arch and the toes. For example, a common structural problem is Morton's foot, in which the first metatarsal is abnormally short and hypermobile. This condition can create biomechanical instabilities of the entire foot, with handicapping pain in the

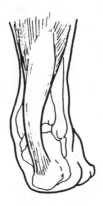

Fig. 4-20. Pronated foot with Helbing's sign.

metatarsal region. Another problem is the fallen metatarsal arch, which can place pressure on the plantar nerve, producing a very painful neuritis along with disability. To alleviate the problem, a special foot pad must be prepared and strategically placed to alleviate the painful pressure and reestablish proper alignment of the metatarsal arch.

Hammer or clawed toes (Fig. 4-21) and crooked toes frequently occur as a result of shoes that are too narrow or too short. For maximum functioning, toes should be maintained in a straight position to efficiently propel the body by pressing or pushing against the supporting base. If the hammer toe or the crooked toe becomes painful, the only alternatives are specialized footwear or surgery to alleviate the diability.

Finally but not least of the toe problems commonly found among dangers are hallux valgus and the tailor's bunion (Fig. 4-22). These problems are the result of shoes or socks that are too short or too narrow, producing abnormal pressure at the metatarsophalangeal joint of the great toe or the little toes. In dancers, the cause may be dancing on pointe before there is adequate strength and joint maturation. In these cases an irritation results, and an extra mineral accumulation occurs in the joint along with toe distortion,

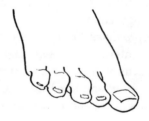

Fig. 4-21. Clawed and hammer toes.

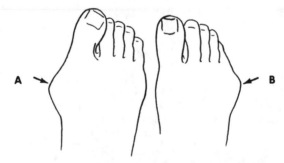

Fig. 4-22. Bunions. A, Hallux valgus. B, Tailor's bunion.

which in the great toe is away from and in the little toe is toward the midline of the body. Early detection of these problems is necessary, combined with proper precautions, to prevent further irritation and deformity. Hallux valgus may also result from stress that is imposed by walking with the hips outward rotated combined with feet that are pronated, whereas the tailor's bunion may stem from hips that are inwardly rotated and feet that are supinated. The dancer must strive at all times to perform straight "tracking" of the leg and foot in locomotion.

Dancers often ask about the value of wearing street shoes with negative heels, or heels that are lower than the soles of the shoes. Many dancers believe that such shoes keep the heel cord stretched out and improve posture. For some individuals, negative-heel shoes present no problems; for others they can cause severe foot and low back pain. Frankly, I believe that they accentuate the problem of the hyperextended knee and force a normally aligned pelvis into malalignment. Another type of sandal that is common to the dancer is one that has a rigid last, often made of wood and having indentations to approximate the positions of the toes. Many dancers who wear these shoes indicate that they cause the toes to grip while walking, therefore increasing the strength of the plantar aspect of the foot, especially the longitudinal arch. This may be true for some individuals; however, the dancer must remember that the foot is not constructed primarily as a gripping device but to push downward against a supporting surface, thereby propelling the body over a terrain. Constant toe gripping while walking may disrupt the basic mechanics of the foot as well as encourage the condition of clawed toes.

Good posture is essential to the dancer in preventing injuries. Good postural alignment reflects muscles that are in balance and functioning efficiently. Constant malalignment and faulty body positioning produce imbalances in opposing musculature. If this occurs over a long period, the supporting and moving structures become chronically imbalanced. In such situations the tissues in and about the area of imbalance are often not able to withstand the rigors of physical stress.

MORPHOLOGIC VARIATIONS IN FEMALE AND MALE DANCERS

It is obvious that there are great variances and dissimilarities in body morphology between male and female. The most common description of body morphology is the somatotype of *endomorph, mesomorph*, and *ectomorph*. The endomorph characteristically is obese, usually having little muscle tone with small bones, large head, long trunk, short neck, and short arms and legs with tapering digits. The endomorph also has sparse, fine hair as well as soft, smooth skin. The mesomorph has a well-defined skeletal structure with strong and highly toned muscles, a broad, sloping shoulder line and a slender waist, wide hips and long arms and legs. The ectomorph, in contrast, has a very thin and narrow build with little muscle tone and long, underdeveloped arms and legs, usually with oversized hands and feet.

Most individuals are mixtures of the three types of body build. The female build is less apt to fit one of them than is the male. The female body form is more mixed, or dysplastic, than the male; however, any body can be altered or modified to some extent through physical training from one body build type to another. Obviously there are movement performance advantages and disadvantages in having a certain somatotype. The most physically versatile somatotype is the mesomorph because of the ability to engage successfully in a great variety of physical activities. Least of these three types in terms of performance expectation is the endomorph. The problem of obesity combined with little muscle tone and strength makes the variety of movements necessary in dance more difficult. It is important that dancers understand their own personal somatotype characteristics so that they can adjust or modify dance activities when necessary. Exceeding limitations of a particular body type may lead to serious injury, and the setting of unrealistic goals based on body type ideals that cannot be achieved may result in discouragement and eventual heartache.

Logically, performance expectations differ for men and women. In general, the male is characteristically stronger than the female but usually has less balance because of his higher center of gravity. Greater strength in the male is due to the greater amount of the hormone testosterone that is secreted in the bloodstream. The female generally is weaker than the male and has a broader and shallower pelvis and a greater angle of the elbow. In the female pelvis there is a more acute hip angle, which produces less mechanical strength advantage in executing running and jumping activities. In activities that involve the arms, such as throwing or supporting the body, the female is usually at a disadvantage because her shoulders are narrower than those of the typical male and because she has a greater angle of the arm at the elbow, which provides less mechanical advantage. One the other hand, the mature female normally has a lower center of gravity than the male; therefore, she has a greater potential for balance and stability.

Research points out that the male and female can work equally hard in physical activities without adverse effects. Contrary to past thinking, exercise is as beneficial to the girl or woman as to the boy or man. A girl should not fear the problem of developing unsightly bulging muscles from vigorous exercise programs. As a rule, the softer fat contours of the female will tend to mask muscle definition stemming from exercise. With proper stretching and equal exercise of antagonist muscles, this type of overdevelopment can be avoided. It is suggested that after performance of a movement pattern that contracts one set of muscles, a pattern should be executed that uses the opposite set of muscles.

An additional factor that must be considered in the female dancer is her menstrual period. Although it was thought in the past that exercise should be avoided during the menstrual period, research now points out that vigorous activity usually causes no ill effects. Medical authorities suggest than when the womb is heavily engorged with blood during the first days of the menstrual period it is advisable to avoid jarring or sudden torque (twisting) movements.

5

The dancer's body

Through proper training over a long period the dancer develops a body that can withstand many physical stresses. A well-conditioned dancer will have stronger bones, ligaments, and muscles than a more sedentary nondancer and as a result will more easily adjust to the torques and shocks imposed by a particular dance form. However, even highly conditioned and skilled dancers may be predisposed to injury by adverse mechanical forces such as abnormal angles of muscle pull, misalignment of body parts, a sudden forceful twist, or a breakdown in the normal synergy of a muscle or muscle group.[14] Dancers often injure themselves as a result of striking improper or unnatural postures. They often attempt movements that are either beyond their particular capabilities or are inappropriate to their particular body build. Because dance is the epitome of motor control and physical endurance, inability to effectively extend oneself over a long period with good body mechanics eventually leads the dancer to sustain an acute or chronic injury.

As in all physically strenuous activities, dance has inherent dangers that can lead to an injury for even the most cautious person. Poor timing, a faulty lift, and a poorly designed stage set are common factors contributing to dance injuries. On and off the stage, the well-trained dancer moves with grace and poise that show efficient positioning of all segments of the body. Every form of dance requires good form and technique. Faulty technique and body placement eventually result in muscle strain, a tendency toward joint sprain, and an inability to effectively withstand chronic stresses applied to the body.

The young and physically immature dancer often trains improperly or attempts movements that are beyond his or her individual maturity level.

The teacher of dance must instruct children at their maturity level. Of particular concern is the fact that children's bones have not finished ossifying, and growth centers can be damaged by unusually severe stress. As with the more physically mature dancer, children can develop pathological conditions affecting their joints and muscles from activities that are beyond their development and maturity levels.

Dance in itself develops positive mental and physical attributes; however, the rigors of dance can countermand these effects. All human beings vary in their basic constitutional strengths based on their inherited physiques. Just as some individuals inherit organic susceptibilities to various diseases such as heart disease or visual problems, individuals inherit peculiarities in body structure that may or may not decrease their ability to withstand physical stresses. Often the dancer's awareness of a potential physical weakness can be dealt with positively by employing better conditioning methods and avoiding activities that may aggravate or prolong the problem.

SITUATIONS THAT MAY CAUSE INJURY

Countless situations in dance may lead to injury; however, there are some that seem to characterize many dance forms and continually create problems for the dancer. The reasons some of these major techniques and/or exercises can create major problems are discussed here.

Turn-out. The turn-out position (Fig. 5-1), in which the dancer stands with the feet in the first position, or at 180 degrees, must be acquired gradually. Primary adjustment must occur within the hips. A student who forces the feet to turn while the knees rotate inward may create the problem of tibial torsion, misaligning the kneecaps and causing a pathological condition on the articular surfaces of the patella. The student should note that the feet should be turned out only if the thigh, kneecap, and foot can be maintained in good alignment.

Plié. Both the demi-plié and the grand plié (Fig. 5-2) must be performed with each body segment properly balanced over the part below. In other words, the back is maintained in a straight position, directly in line with the pelvis and hip, which are, in turn, in line with the thigh, kneecap, lower leg, and foot. Pliés performed incorrectly can produce severe stress on the inner aspects of the knee, perhaps accentuating or even causing knock-knees, promoting the pronated foot, and lowering the inner longitudinal arch of the foot.

Lifting a partner overhead. When lifting a partner overhead (Fig. 5-3), the male must keep his partner as close to his center of gravity as possible.

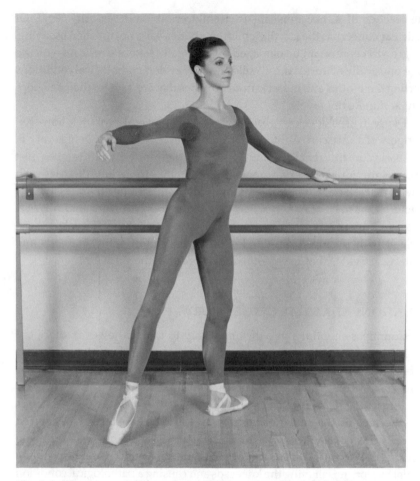

Fig. 5-1. The turn-out, if forced, can lead to serious leg problems.

The female dancer's center of gravity and body weight fall in a straight line along the balanced posture of her male partner. To avoid back strain, the male must also keep his body in good alignment by keeping the back relatively straight and the pelvis positioned directly under the trunk.

Lifting a partner from the floor. A basic rule for lifting a bulky or heavy object is that the point of support should be positioned as nearly as possible over or under the center of the object to be lifted. The primary lifting force should be initiated by the legs with the knees bent and the back held as straight as possible (Fig. 5-4). Violating this rule results in much more energy expended than is necessary and places injurious strain on the lifter's lower back.

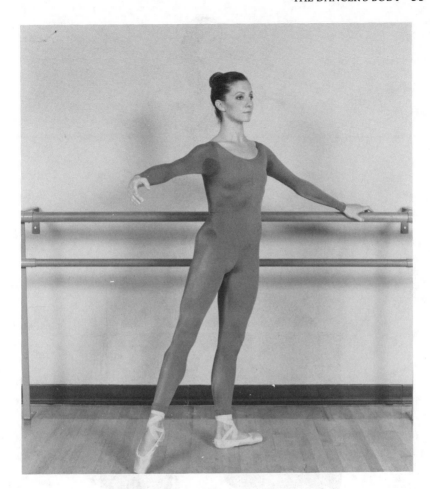

Fig. 5-1, cont'd. For legend see opposite page.

Landing from a jump. Stress from landing (Fig. 5-5) is less when the head, trunk, and legs are properly aligned. In this manner, shock is transmitted equally along the outer length of the spine, starting at the feet and ending at the base of the head.

Second position in air to arabesques. The second position in air to arabesques (a'la seconde en l'air) (Fig. 5-6) are techniques that place a great deal of strain on the hip joint. To avoid unnecessary stress, the performer must hold the trunk erect and keep the supporting leg straight at all times, with the pelvis and trunk in as correct alignment as possible. In the movement the dancer must avoid overarching the lower back. Incorrect technique can lead to lower back and hip problems.

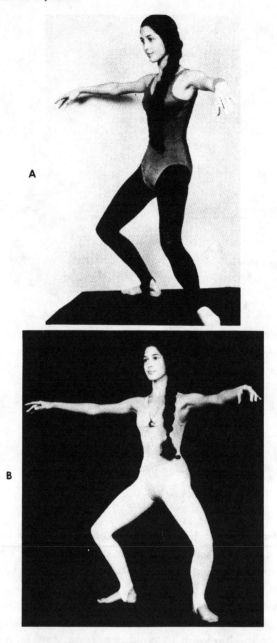

Fig. 5-2. Plie in second position. **A,** Incorrect positioning. Abnormal stress is placed on the inside of the feet, ankles, knees, and hips. The shoulders and lower back do not form a straight line over the legs. **B,** Correct positioning. Each body segment is well balanced over the part below. Knees are over feet. Weight is distributed evenly over entire foot.

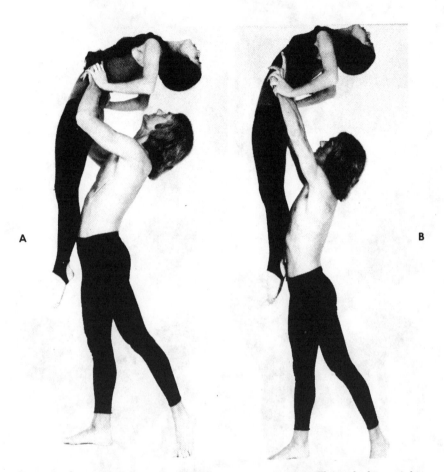

Fig. 5-3. Lifting a partner overhead. **A,** Incorrect positioning. The male dancer is leaning back too far, failing to properly distribute the weight of the female along his posture line. Abnormal stress is produced in the male dancer's neck and lower back. **B,**
Correct positioning. This lift is executed with the smallest amount of strain possible.
The female dancer's center of gravity and body weight fall in a straight line along the
balanced posture of the male dancer.

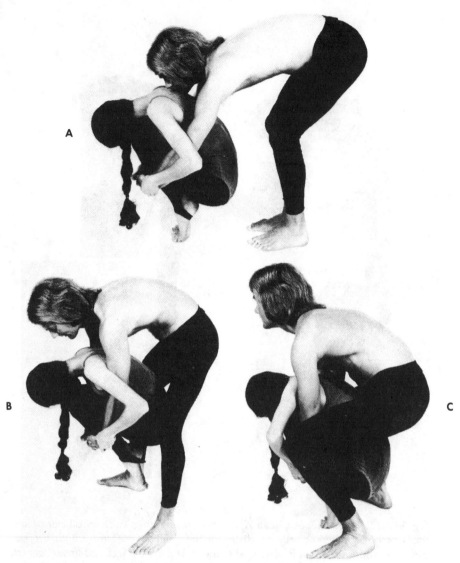

Fig. 5-4. Lifting a partner from the floor. **A,** Incorrect positioning. The female dancer is positioned too far out from her partner's center of gravity, placing unnecessary stress on the male dancer's lower back. **B,** Incorrect positioning. The position of the male is better here than in **A.** However, it is still injury producing because his back is rounded, his knees are too straight, and the weight of the partner is in front of his center of gravity. **C,** Correct positioning. The position in **C** is less injury producing than either **A** or **B** because the head of the male dancer is raised, the back is straighter, the knees are bent, and the major weight of the female dancer is more directly under the hips of her partner. In this initial position the lift is mainly executed by the strength of the thighs, placing little stress on the back and shoulders.

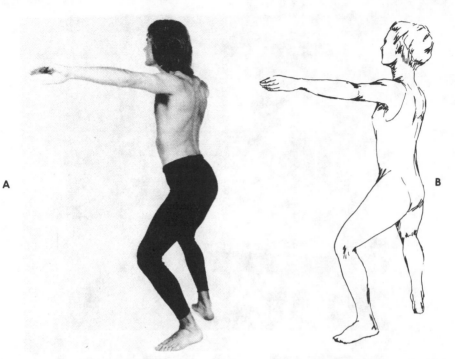

Fig. 5-5. Landing from a second position jump. A, Incorrect positioning. The shock of landing is not distributed equally along the entire length of the dancer's body. Knees are not positioned over the center of the feet, lower back is arched, and head is thrust forward. **B,** Correct positioning. Stress of landing is less when the head, trunk, and legs are correctly aligned. Shock is transmitted equally along the outer length of the spine, starting at the feet and ending at the base of the head.

Passé (Retiré). One leg is drawn up the length of the lower leg until the toes are positioned back of the other knee. When held as a pose it is called retiré. Segmental alignment is necessary to avoid adverse hip stress (Fig. 5-7).

Foot and ankle placement. As with all body segments, the foot and ankle must be kept in good alignment (Fig. 5-8). This is particularly true when one is performing a relevé to a demi-pointe or a full pointe (Fig. 5-9). When one moves to a position on the balls of the feet, it is essential that all five toes help to maintain support and that the fore-, mid-, and hindfoot sections are in direct line with the lower leg and kneecap. A violation of proper foot alignment can place abnormal strain not only on the arches of the foot but also on knees, hips, and back.

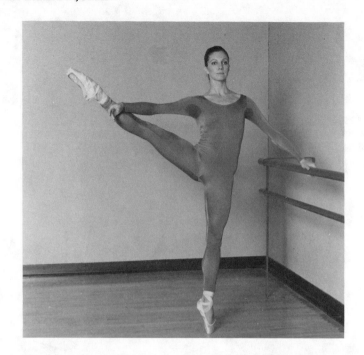

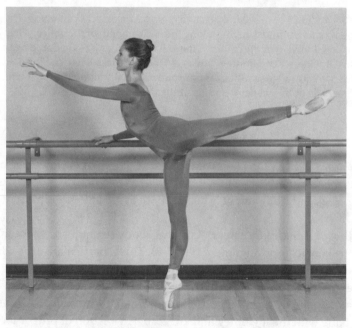

Fig. 5-6. A, The grand battement and **B,** arabesque, if improperly executed, can create serious hip problems.

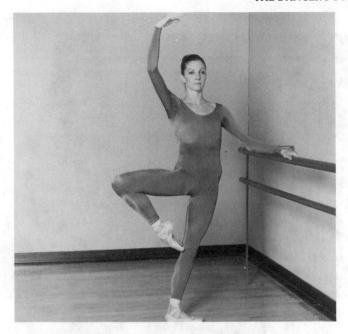

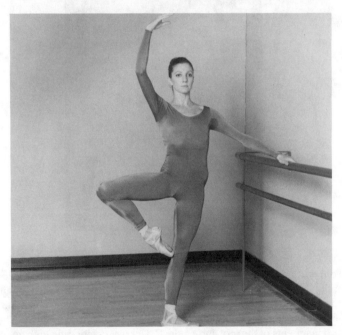

Fig. 5-7. Passé (Retiré). **A,** Incorrect positioning. Misalignment causes adverse hip stress and awkward gripping of the barre. **B,** Correct positioning. The dancer pulls "out of her hip," seeming taller, with an extended arm gently resting on the barre.

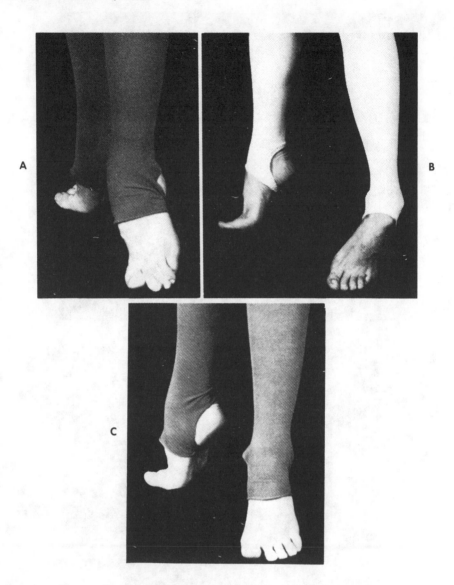

Fig. 5-8. Foot and ankle placement. **A,** Incorrect positioning with sickling in. Sickling in , or eversion and pronation of the foot and ankle, causes strain on the longitudinal arch and the great toe and tends to roll the heel outward. **B,** Incorrect positioning with sickling out. Inversion, or a rolling inward of the foot, places great strain on the outer tendons and ligaments of the foot and ankle. **C,** Correct positioning with good lower limb placement. The toes are, for the most part, straight and flat on the supporting surface as well as properly aligned with the forefoot. The forefoot forms a straight line to the midfoot, the back of the foot, and the lower leg.

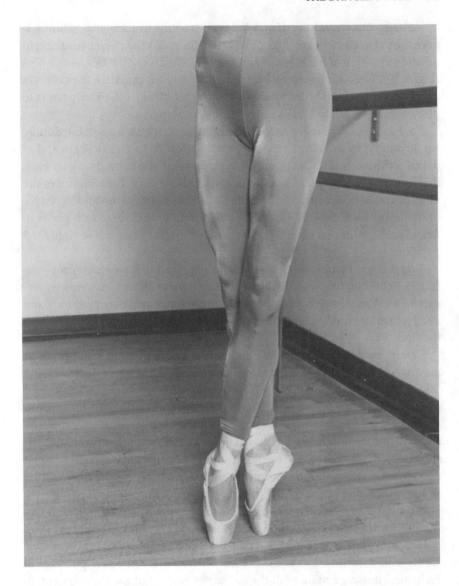

Fig. 5-9. Foot and leg alignment is extremely important while on pointe.

Sitting in a stretch position. While one is sitting in a stretch position, it is necessary that the feet and legs be in direct line with the pelvis, resulting in equal contraction of the internal and external muscles of the thighs and hips (Fig. 5-10). Keeping the spine in a straight line helps maintain the pelvis in good alignment with both the trunk and thighs. Sitting incorrectly tends to place abnormal strain on the inner thighs and hips.

Sit-ups and double leg lifts. Both the straight leg sit-up and the double leg lift should be avoided as exercises to develop abnormal strength and as dance techniques (Fig. 5-11). Each places extreme strain on the lower back that can subsequently lead to chronic back problems. In both instances the iliopsoas muscle is contracted, forcing the accentuation of the lordotic curve of the lower back. Sit-ups should be performed with one or both knees in flexed position, or one but not both legs may be lifted while in a straightened position.

Back arch. Hyperextending the back may lead to lower back problems (Fig. 5-12). At no time should the beginning dancer attempt extreme hyperextension. A good rule of thumb to follow in extension of the upper back and head is to maintain the abdomen, pelvis, and thighs in a flattened position on the floor.

Deep knee bend. Forcefully bending the knees in a full squat position may overly stretch internal ligaments of the knee joint (cruciate ligaments) (Fig. 5-13). This is especially true for dancers with large thighs. In a full squat position the knee is forced open; this is increased when there is extra bulk in the backs of the thighs. It is desirable that the full squat be gradually conditioned and that the heavy-thighed individual avoid the technique completely. It should also be noted that the beginner should never engage in ballistic squat movements. The demi-plié and the grand plié, when performed correctly, should place little strain on the integrity of the knee.

Ballistic movements. "Ballistic" implies a rebounding movement employing an alternate contraction of opposing muscles or groups of muscles. Ballistic movements can be divided into two types: controlled and uncontrolled. Controlled ballistic movements are initiated by a conscious application of reciprocal muscle action, with the dancer in control of each movement. In uncontrolled ballistic movements, the dancer lunges or slams into another body part without consciously controlling the action. The uncontrolled movement is more likely to injure ligaments and joints and to tear muscles. No matter what his or her level of ability, every dancer must gradually lead up to performing ballistic movements by making sure that the body is thoroughly warmed up.

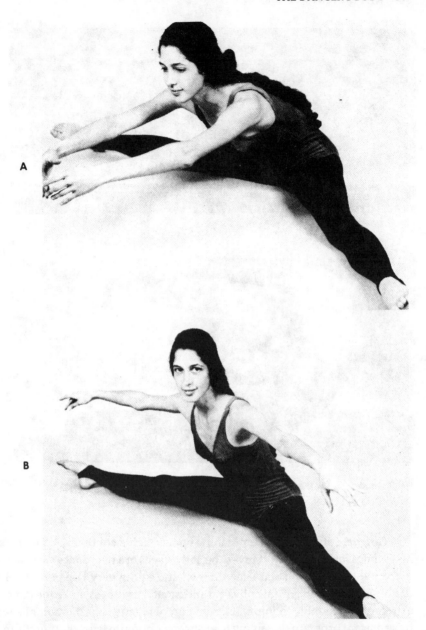

Fig. 5-10. Sitting stretch in second position. **A,** Incorrect positioning. Dancer is rolling the hip and thigh inward and rounding the upper back. In this faulty position, strain may occur to the groin and inner thigh. **B,** Correct positioning. Injury is not likely because the legs and feet are in a straight line with the pelvis, resulting in equal contraction of the internal and external muscles of the hip. Extending the spine maintains the pelvis in good alignment with both the trunk and thighs.

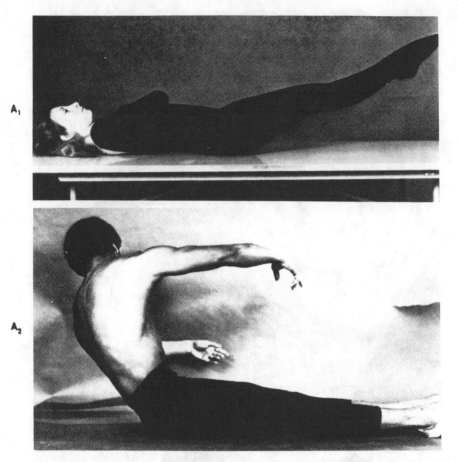

Fig. 5-11. A, Double leg lifts and straight leg sit-ups place abnormal stress on the dancer's lower back.

Fatigue. Fatigue is a factor that the dancer fights continually. The most likely times for injuries to occur are the early stages of a new dance experience when the body is not adequately trained and in the very late periods of a dance session when chronic physical and mental tiredness make the dancer extremely vulnerable to injury. Elimination of fatigue is best accomplished by a constant program of training to ensure an optimum level of strength and flexibility combined with muscular and cardiovascular endurance.

THE DANCER'S ENVIRONMENT

While the relationship between dance injuries and particular techniques and practices is strong, one should never discount the dancer's

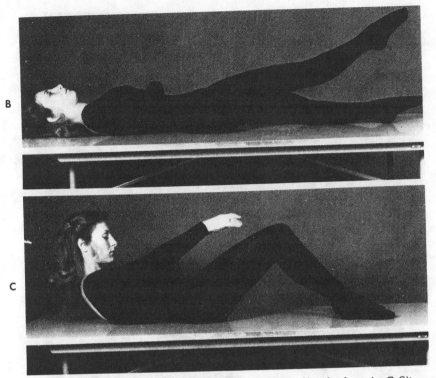

Fig. 5-11, cont'd. B, Single leg lifts reduce the possibility of low back strain. **C,** Sit-ups should be performed with the back rounded and the knees bent.

environs. In other words, everything that surrounds dancers, including the clothing as well as the practice hall and performance hall, can directly or indirectly cause injury.

Clothing. In general, the costume that the dancer wears for practice or for the actual performance is not usually dangerous unless it perhaps is ill suited for the part. Cumbersome or bulky clothing should be avoided, especially when a certain dance technique may result in tripping or in a limb getting caught in the fabric and becomed strained (Fig. 5-14). Proper footwear is of the great concern to the dancer. When one considers that as many as seven pairs of ballet slippers may be used by a professional ballerina in just one week, the importance of proper support is clear. In a given performance, a dancer may alternate between pointe shoes, classical slippers, and jazz shoes, all of which must fit appropriately as well as provide support. Most hazards to feet are compounded when the dancer works without any foot covering or wears slippers that offer little protection.[21] When not dancing,

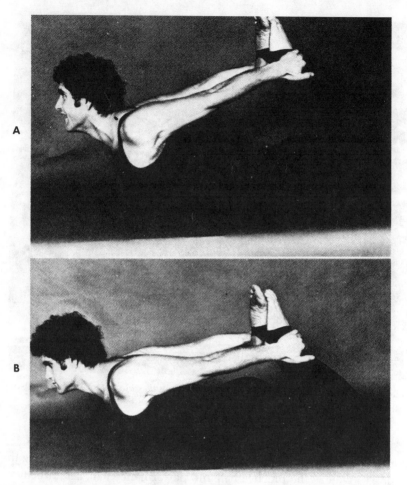

Fig. 5-12. A, Hyperextending the back may lead to low back strain. **B,** Low back injury can be reduced if the dancer maintains the hips and lower abdomen in contact with the supporting surface.

the dancer should wear street shoes that provide good support, particularly when standing or walking on a nonyielding surface such as cement.

The dance surface. Dancers must continually adjust to their environment. The dance environments of the stage and studio present tremendous demands on the body and emotions as a dancer adjusts to variations in area, size, and surface resistance. Stage surfaces can accentuate the problems of the dancer's fatigue. Ideally the dance surface should have resiliency, yielding to the force of the dancer's body. Dancing on a rigid nonyielding surface overtaxes

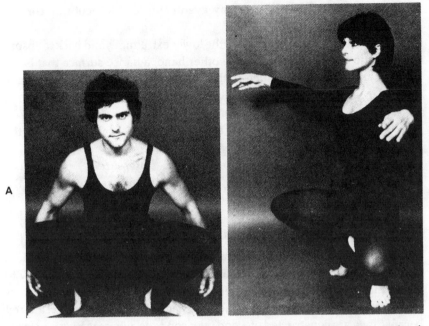

Fig. 5-13. A full squat may cause knee ligament injury, especially if the full weight of the dancer forces a sudden opening of the knee joint.

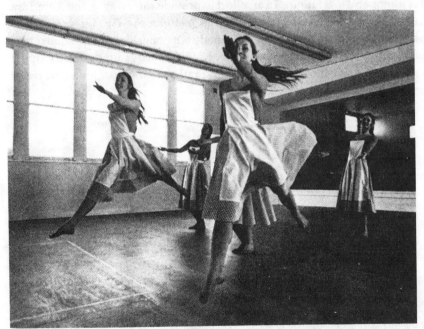

Fig. 5-14. A dancer's clothing should not be bulky or cumbersome.

tensons, joints, and bones and may eventually lead to acute or chronic pathological conditions.

A surface that is too firm causes the lower extremities and back to absorb much of the impact energy. On the other hand, a dance surface that is too resilient and absorbs too much of the impact energy leads to early fatigue in the dancer.[22] In general, dance floors should:*

1. Have shock-absorbing qualities
2. Be resilient to some degree and at the same time absorb some of the impact forces
3. Not permanently deform or dent under pressure
4. Not be dead or yield softly like sand, but must return some of the bounce to the dancer's shoe
5. Not be bouncy as with a trampoline
6. Not be absolutely hard or rigid

Dancing on a different type of surface each day, such as a highly resilient stage one day and unyielding cement the next, does not allow the body to adapt and may create chronic stress that eventually may result in stress fractures or joint degeneration. American stages have often been criticized because they are constructed of wood over concrete, whereas Russian stages are constructed by placing wood over an air space, allowing for more effortless jumps and less fatigue. In an effort to provide safer stages, the American Guild of Musical Artists and the United Institute for Theater Technology have suggested that floor surfaces be made out of northern maple laid over a matrix of two-by-four cross beams.[25] Traveling dance groups should employ a portable floor with soft underpadding rather than dance on concrete or asphalt.

---

*Adapted from Snell, F.D., Inc., Discussion of test results in Snell Report on Resilient Factors of Different Flooring Construction to Maple Flooring Manufacturers Association., Feb. 1966, New York, F.D. Snell, Inc.

III

MAJOR FACTORS IN INJURY PREVENTION

In Part III, three areas of injury prevention have been selected as being of major importance to the dancer; namely, preparing the body, nutrition, and psychological factors. Each area is unique and discrete yet interrelated.

6

Preparing the body to prevent injury

One of the most important factors in dance is the preparation of the body to withstand the rigors of physical stress. It is essential that a dancer know his or her body requirements to the extent that conditioning exercises become selective. In other words, not every individual has the same exercise needs. Needs will differ based on a body build, heredity, prior experience, past injuries, particular dance form engaged in, and the level of ability attained in dance. A generalization can be made, however, that every dancer must have an appropriate degree of strength, joint flexibility, and muscular and cardiovascular endurance as well as coordination. This chapter is an overview of the most pertinent aspects of the key areas of physical conditioning as they relate to the dancer and provides selected exercises specifically designed to condition the areas of the body that dancers injure most often.

STRENGTH

Strength is the most important physiological factor in the prevention of dancer injuries. It is defined as the capacity of the individual to exert a muscle contraction or force against a resistance. When muscles are regularly exercised, important physiological changes, as well as an increase in muscle girth or size, take place. However, for a muscle to develop size and strength it must be stressed by progressive overloading.

For example, an individual can engage in an increased number of repetitions of a particular movement and produce strength up to a point. This

73

type of exercise, however, will increase only the dancer's ability to sustain a specific movement rather than increase strength. Other means of overloading can be applied by gradually increasing a resistance to a specific muscle or group of muscles.

Strength may be identified by two subdivisions, namely, dynamic and static strength. *Dynamic* strength is the ability of the individual to overcome resistance through a complete range of movement, and it can be divided into isotonic and isokinetic strength. *Isotonic* strength is defined as application of a range of movement against a constant resistance. *Isokinetic* strength is defined as application of a full range of movement while the involved muscle group contracts maximally at a constant speed and varies in or accommodates the resistance according to the strength of that specific muscle group. A second type of strength (used very little in dance) is *isometric*, or static, strength, which is the ability to apply resistance against an immovable force.

Because strength in general allows the dancer to move freely and handle the body efficiently, it also plays an extremely important role in the prevention of injury. However, for strength to be most effective it must be properly balanced between the agonist and antagonist muscles. Therefore, a dancer concerned with injury prevention should be concerned with general muscle development, avoiding overdeveloping strength of specific muscle groups.

Over the years, dancers have resisted engaging in strength overload programs such as weight lifting. Recently an increased number of dancers are participating in specific programs of strength development employing both non-equipment and equipment approaches.

Non-equipment approaches include calisthenic or free-type exercise or partner and self-resistance. In most cases isotonic movements are employed. In the case of free-type exercise, the dancer and the body weight usually act as a resistance against gravity.

By exercising with a partner, both strength and flexibility can markedly increase. This type of exercise requires partners of about equal size and strength and is performed much like isokinetic exercise with accommodating resistance occurring through a complete range of motion. All types of movements can be engaged in using this method. The body part to be exercised is taken into a stretched position by the partner. Resistance is applied and accommodated through a complete range of motion. Three bouts of isokinetic resistance are employed for each exercise.

Equipment approaches for increasing strength are almost too numerous to mention. They range from free weights such as dumbells and barbells to pulley devices or machine resistance devices such as Nautilus machines.

One system that employs both resistance and dance movement patterns is the Pilates System. Developed in the early 1900s by Joseph Pilates, it came to the United States from Europe in the 1930s. The exercise system employs mat exercises as well as specialized equipment exercises. One major piece of equipment is called the Universal reformer (Fig. 6-1), which is a horizontal platform with a movable carriage on which the dancer reclines, sits, or stands. Resistance is controlled by four detachable springs. The Pilates System is used as a method of conditioning, but also for rehabilitation following an injury. This approach helps the dancer increase or restore strength, flexibility and movement patterns necessary in a particular dance form such as ballet or modern.

FLEXIBILITY

Flexibility is one of the dancer's most important concerns. Flexibility can be defined in many different ways, but in essence it is the amplitude of joint movement or the extent to which a limb can be extended and flexed. There are many causes for a decrease or increase in flexibility: anatomical, physiological, or even emotional. The human body varies greatly in its ability to engage in a broad spectrum of movement. One such variation is in the dancer's joint structure. A person who has a heavy skeletal formation may not be able to engage in a full range of movement activity as can an individual

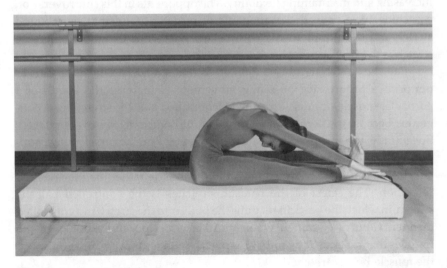

Fig. 6-1. Universal reformer.

who has a lighter or more delicate design. On the other hand, joints may differ according to their ligamentous organization. A joint that is heavily bound by ligaments may be more restricted than a lightly supported joint. Bulky musculature and tight, unyielding tendons can also restrict range of movement. Because one muscle is relaxed while an opposing muscle is contracted, the dancer can consciously "let go" of a part; this is commonly called reciprocal coordination. Although most restricted movements of joints and limbs are of an anatomical or physiological origin, a person's mental and emotional characteristics have a great deal to do with the ability to relax. The tense individual who apears restricted and withdrawn because of painful emotions often reflects these feelings in a rigid and unyielding body.

One must be reminded that posture affects the pliability and extensibility of the body's musculature. When considering flexibility, one must also remember that the habitual positions that one takes in life can alter joint range of motion. The more sedentary people are, the less able they are to perform a variety of movements. Very active people, on the other hand, who engage in a variety of different activities throughout the day will usually be more flexible than their less-active peers.

Increasing joint range of movement

In recent years there has been much discussion as to the best method of increasing and maintaining flexibility. The opponents in this controversy on stretching have been the proponents of ballistic (bouncing) or rebound stretch and those individuals who believe that static or gradual increase stretch is the best approach.

Ballistic stretching can be defined as that stretch in which the dancer performs a progressive pulsating movement to increase the length of a particular muscle or muscle group. Uncontrolled ballistic stretching is dangerous, because the performer often allows the body part to be overstretched. Specifically, the uncontrolled ballistic movement can adversely affect supporting ligaments and may result in muscle strain by accentuating the myotatic reflex, causing a contraction within the muscle rather than the desired relaxation. The safest of the ballistic stretches is the controlled ballistic stretch, in which the participant pulls the body into the stretch in a controlled manner. Control is gained when the dancer purposefully thinks of the muscles that pull the body into the stretch and those that are antagonistic to the muscle being stretched.

The static or gradual stretch differs from the ballistic type in that the performer takes the desired position of stretch, pulls the body to the point where it can no longer go, and then gradually tries to pull past this positioin for 30 seconds to 1 minute. In the first phase of the gradual stretch the dancer assumes the stretch position and then relaxes in that position for 20 to 30 seconds. Relaxed, the dancer then slowly extends into the actual stretch, extending for about 30 seconds. In the second phase, as with the controlled ballistic stretch, the dancer concentrates on the muscles that pull him or her into the stretch. Also, while at the resistance point the performer should force all air from the lungs, allowing the stretch to be increased, sometimes as much as 2 to 6 inches.

The controlled ballistic and the static stretch have been found to be equally effective in increasing range of movement; however, ballistic stretch tends to aggravate muscle tissue, and small muscle tears and spasms may occur, discouraging the performer in attempts to further engage in activity. Static or gradual stretching tends to decrease the tendency toward muscle spasm and muscle soreness in the very early states of activity. Consequently, gradual stretch is preferred, particularly in the very early stages of a conditioning program.

In essence, stretching exercises are most effective when executed slowly and deliberately rather than with bouncing or jerking movements. Ballistic movements tend to stimulate the stretch reflex and, in some cases, overly tense muscles instead of producing relaxation, making them vulnerable to spasms and tearing.

A third technique of stretching is fast becoming popular among dancers. This technique uses the concept of muscle relaxation through stimulation of the proprioceptors.[15] This approach uses the physiological fact that a muscle contraction is normally followed by relaxation of the opposite antagonist muscle. One method applicable to dance is to forcibly contract one set of muscles against a resistance and then immediately begin a gradual stretch of the opposing muscle group. For example, the dancer extends the lower leg several times against a resistance, such as a fellow dancer's hand or a wall (contracting the quadriceps muscles as much as possible), and immediately follows with a gradual (static) stretch of the hamstring group. This same procedure could be applied in any body areas. If the application of a resistance is impractical or difficult, the dancer can still facilitate stimulation by three or four quick isotonic (no resistance) contractions of the opposing muscle followed by a stretch.

MANAGING MUSCULAR SORENESS AND STIFFNESS

Many theories exist as to why active people develop muscle soreness following physical activity. A common belief is that delayed soreness develops in muscles as a result of minute muscle spasms and perhaps even small muscle tears; however, recent research indicates that this problem may be related to the disruption of the connective tissue elements in muscles and/or their attachments.[1] This may cause a mild inflammation in the muscle, with resultant pain caused by the pressure of swelling on pain receptors. Soreness often follows unaccustomed physical activity. Stiffness is associated with the same circumstances as muscle soreness; however, its cause is not as apparent as that of soreness. In cases of either muscular soreness or stiffness, the dancer complains of a decrease in muscle tissue extensibility and limb flexibility.

One method of helping to overcome muscle soreness and stiffness is to follow a program of gradual stretching at the beginning of an intense exercise period and to follow up with the same stretching regimen at the end of the class. Stretching at the end of class helps to reduce muscle tension. This procedure is best followed by about 2 weeks in a new class or routine situation. After the 2-week period has passed, the body has become accustomed to using different muscles and may require only a gradual stretching regimen at the beginning of the class session or actual performance.

The amplitude of joint movement is specific to the types of activities that are habitually engaged in, and each person has his or her own flexibility characteristics. It is important that the dancer eliminate the possibility of sudden strain or twist by being as flexible as possible. However, joint range of movement should not be developed at the expense of a balance of strength. One should note that a joint that is too lax is prone to dislocation or degenerative disease, and a muscle that is too tight is prone to muscle strain.

STAMINA

Stamina is the staying power of the body in a given activity or activities and may be divided into two basic components: muscle endurance and cardiovascular endurance. Muscle endurance is the ability of the dancer to sustain many muscle contractions over a given period. Muscle endurance cannot be separated from muscle strength because it is part of a continuum. The dancer's muscle endurance is of the utmost importance to sustain a high quality of movement for a long period.

Because dancing can be one of the most grueling of endeavors, requiring many hours dedicated to practice, the efficiency of the heart and lungs—the cardiovascular system—is an inseparable component of the dancer's physical fitness. The body cannot be used effectively as a tool for creative expression without all physical fitness factors being at the highest level possible. The ability to effectively deliver oxygen to the muscle tissue over a long period demands a strong and efficient cardiorespiratory system. To produce an oxygen delivery system that is efficient and able to withstand the rigors of long hours of physical activity, the heart muscle must be strong. In the well-conditioned heart muscle, each contraction places a greater than average volume of blood into the general circulation. As the heart becomes trained it also beats fewer times per minute. Training sometimes reduces the pulse rate as much as 10 to 20 beats per minute as efficiency increases. The well-conditioned heart also returns to its normal beat much more quickly than the poorly-conditioned heart and recuperates more quickly from physical fatigue. Because of the better transportation of oxygen to all the body's tissue, the products of metabolism are more quickly removed. The trained respiratory system is able to handle oxygen more efficiently; consequently, there is an increased use of oxygen. The trained dancer with an efficient cardiovascular system is able to endure a high level of physical performance for a long period without the distress of physical fatigue.

To improve efficiency of the heart and lungs, the overload principle must be employed as it is in improving strength. Cardiovascular endurance, therefore, can be increased as the dancer forces the body to engage in activity over a long period, gradually increasing the rate and intensity of training. While not participating in dance, the dancer should engage in different types of sustained activity such as bicycling, jogging, and, to a lesser degree, swimming. A good subjective indication of increasing cardiovascular fitness is a pulse rate that becomes slower as training progresses. Dancers, as a group, tend to ignore cardiovascular conditioning; however, the serious dancer should be extremely concerned with the efficiency of the cardiovascular system.

WARMING UP AND COOLING DOWN

The importance of warm-up has been debated for many decades; it is still considered unnecessary by some authorities. I, along with the vast majority of trained movement professionals, consider proper warm-up to be a necessary prelude to dancing. Bodily movement is the most effective means of warming up. Research has determined that the use of such warm-up procedures as massage, use of analgesic balms, and hot showers have little positive effect on performance. There is, however, vast disagreement as to how much and what type of activity is necessary to adequately warm-up the performer. In general, the primary purpose of a warm-up before vigorous physical activity is to raise the deep temperatures within the body and to elongate contracted ligaments and fascia as well as musculature. If these factors are taken into consideration, the body is then able to withstand the various rigors of intensive physical activity. Research has also shown that proper warm-up increases the speed of nerve impulse transmission.

A proper warm-up, depending on the activity to be engaged in and the vigor that the activity demands, should last from 10 to 20 or even 30 minutes, until perspiration is apparent and the body has been fully stretched. (The older dancer needs a longer warm-up period than the younger dancer.) Warm-up procedures should range from general to specific movements. The dancer should first be concerned with increasing the heart rate and gradually increasing the deep temperatures of the body. This can be accomplished by easy running or prancing in place or around the studio for 5 to 10 minutes, followed by light general movement of all the joints. When perspiration has broken out on the skin and a feeling of body warmth is experienced, the dancer should then proceed with a stretching routine including either gradual stretch or facilitative techniques or both. Following the stretch phase, the dancer should be concerned with "stylized" warming up, involving the primary movements or combinations that will be used in the dance to be performed. It is extremely important in terms of injury prevention for the dancer to finish the warm-up session with movements from the dance that will be performed. Following this warm-up approach, the body is in a state of readiness: there is an increase in temperature, blood sugar, and adrenalin, and joints are unencumbered in preparation for vigorous activity.

Following vigorous dancing, the dancer should allow the body to gradually cool-down. Circulation should be permitted to slow down gradually, with the heart rate returning to the preexercise level. It is extremely harmful to stop activity while the heart is pumping vigorously. In this situation body fluids tend to pool in the lower limbs, causing extreme discomfort and soreness. Rather than stopping suddenly, the dancer should continue to move for 3 to 5 minutes following activity until the heart rate and breathing have returned to normal. At the end of the cool-down procedure, the dancer should engage in a general stretching routine to reduce muscle tension.[3]

SPECIAL PREVENTIVE EXERCISES

It is not the intention of this chapter to present an extensive discussion of individual exercises that a dancer might perform but to present key exercises selected for their ability to assist in the prevention of specific injuries.

Key stretching exercises

Each stretch should be executed gradually. First, assume the proper position and stretch gently for 20 to 30 seconds, and then proceed to the actual gradual stretch for up to 30 seconds. A stretch should never be executed so vigorously as to cause pain. When the full extent of the stretch has been reached, the dancer should settle further by pushing the air completely out of the lungs. Release from the stretch position should always be done slowly, never quickly.

Calf Stretch (Fig. 6-2)

Purpose. To stretch the heel cord, calf muscle, and back of the leg and to prevent heel cord strain.

Space and/or equipment. Barre, wall, or the back of a chair to support hands.

Starting position. Stand at arm's length from an arm support with the body inclined forward. Extend the leg to be stretched backward with the foot flat on the floor, toes pointing straight ahead.

Execution

1. Allow the body to fall forward slowly, keeping the foot flat at all times. To stretch the soleus muscle bend knee and allow the body to fall forward.
2. Repeat two or three times on each leg.

Variation. Stretch body heel cords at the same time using the above method. Stand on an incline with one heel or both heels lower than the toes.

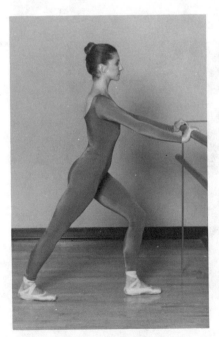 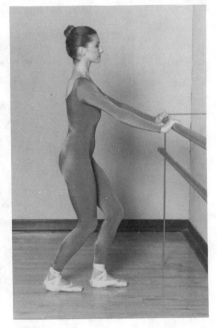

Fig. 6-2. A, Calf stretch. **B,** Calf stretch variation.

Front of Leg Stretch (Fig. 6-3)

Purpose. To stretch the forepart of the lower leg and thigh; assists in the prevention and/or treatment of shin splints.

Space and/or equipment. Firm, but covered, surface and a rolled towel.

Starting position. Sit on the legs with knees together and a rolled towel placed under the extended toes.

Execution

1. Allow full weight to be placed gradually on the lower legs. Return to starting position.
2. Repeat one to three times.

CAUTION: Avoid this exercise if there is a history of knee injury.

Hamstring Stretch (Fig. 6-4)

Purpose. To stretch the hamstring muscle group and the upper attachment of the calf muscle.

Space and/or equipment. Firm exercise mat.

Starting position. Assume a long sitting position with knees perfectly straight and legs together.

Execution

1. From the long sitting position, bend forward from the waist and reach as far forward as possible with the hands.

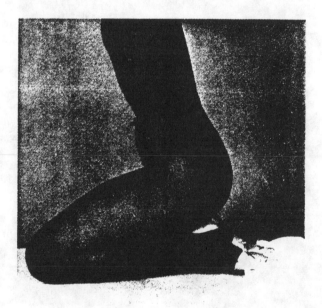

Fig. 6-3. Front of the leg stretch.

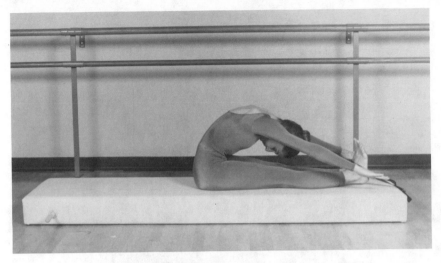

Fig. 6-4. Hamstring stretch.

2. First, stretch with the toes pointed (plantar flexion), placing emphasis on the hamstring muscle group. Then, with the foot pulled back as far as possible (dorsiflexion), emphasize stretching the upper attachment of the calf muscle.

3. Repeat two or three times.

Variation. Stretch as above but progressively widen the distance between the legs.

Stork Stretch (Fig. 6-5)

Purpose. To stretch the quadriceps muscle group, specifically the rectus femoris muscle, which, besides helping to extend the lower leg, acts as a hip flexor, and the iliopsoas muscle, a primary hip flexor; also assists in remediation of lumbar lordosis.

Space and/or equipment. Barre or the back of a straight-backed chair.

Starting position. Standing in good postural alignment, bend the lower leg and grasp the ankle with the hand on the same side.

Execution

1. Keeping the thigh in the same alignment as the support leg, pull the heel of the foot toward the buttocks and then pull the upper leg backward as far as possible without overly arching the lower back.

2. Repeat two or three times.

CAUTION: To avoid placing stress on the lower back, the body must always be maintained in good alignment without arching the lower back.

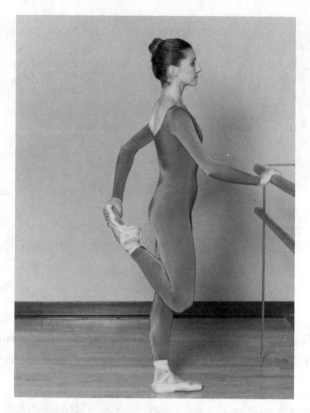

Fig. 6-5. Stork stretch. Standing in a straight line position.

Facedown Thigh and Hip Flexor Stretch (Fig. 6-6)

Purpose. To stretch the quadricips muscle group, specifically the rectus femoris muscle and the iliopsoas hip flexor muscle; may also assist in remediation of lumbar lordosis.

Space and/or equipment. Exercise mat.

Starting position. Lie facedown with the body turned slightly to one side. Bend the leg on the turned side as far as possible and grasp the ankle with the hand on the same side.

Execution

1. Without arching the back, pull the leg as far as possible to the buttocks region and then lift the thigh off of the mat.
2. Repeat two or three times and then change to stretch the other leg.

   CAUTION: Extreme care should be taken not to pull the pelvis back to the extent that the lower back becomes overly arched.

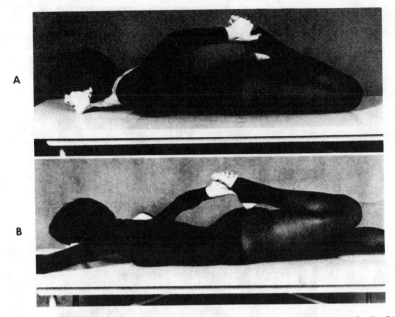

Fig. 6-6. Facedown thigh and hip flexor stretch. **A,** Double leg stretch. **B,** Single leg stretch.

Chair Hip Flexor Stretch (Fig. 6-7)

Purpose. To stretch the hip flexors and to assist in the remediation of forward pelvic tilt and lumbar lordosis.

Space and/or equipment. A chair with a firm seat or a bench.

Starting position. Standing in good alignment 1 or 2 feet from the chair seat or bench, step up so that one foot is on the seat and the other is firmly fixed on the floor. Both feet are facing directly ahead.

Execution

1. Slowly lower the body toward the floor, placing tension on the thigh and hip of the support side.
2. Repeat two or three times and then change sides.

Spine Flattener (Fig. 6-8)

Purpose. To stretch the long extensors of the spine and to assist in the remediation of an abnormal lordotic curve of the neck and lower back.

Space and/or equipment. Floor.

Starting position. Assume a hooklike lying position with the fingertips placed directly under the lower back.

Execution

1. Pull the chin in until the neck curve is straightened as much as

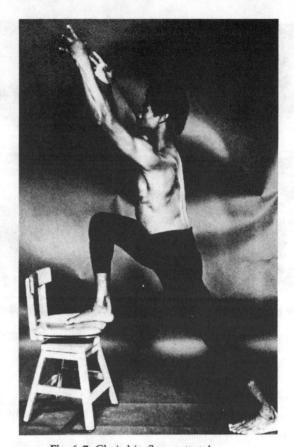

Fig. 6-7. Chair hip flexor stretch.

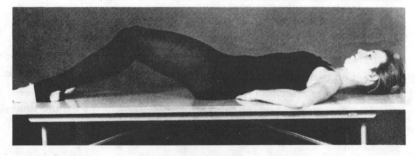

Fig. 6-8. Spine flattener.

possible. Hold this position. Next, flatten the lower back by tightening the abdominal and buttock muscles and press downward until the fingertips feel the pressure of the lower back.

2. While maintaining the neck and back in a flat position, slowly slide the feet forward until the neck and/or the lower back cannot be kept flat.
3. The point at which the back or neck cannot be kept flat is the area that the dancer should concentrate on for increasing muscle extensibility.
4. Repeat two or three times.

Long Stretch of the Upper and Lower Back (Fig. 6-9)

Purpose. To stretch the long extensor muscles of the back with special emphasis on rounding the lower back.

Space and/or equipment. Firm mat.

Starting position. Assume a long lying position with arms fully extended overhead and legs curled over the head.

Execution

1. With legs overhead, slowly attempt to first touch the toes and then the knees to the mat. Round the lower back as much as possible.
2. Execute one time only.

CAUTION: This stretch may place abnormal strain on the neck. Ideally, the body weight should be evenly distributed on the shoulders and head.

Double Knee Rotation (Fig. 6-10)

Purpose. To stretch the lower back.

Space and/or equipment. Firm exercise mat.

Starting position. Assume a hooklike lying position with arms out to the side or across the chest.

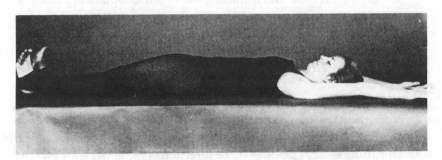

Fig. 6-9. Long stretch of the upper and lower back.

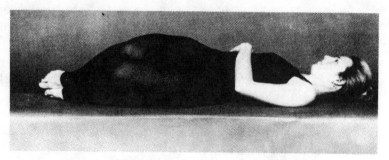

Fig. 6-10. Double knee low back rotation stretch.

Execution
1. Keeping the feet and back flat on the mat, rotate both legs first to one side and then to the other side.
2. Repeat two or three times.

Variation. Change the position of the feet from close to the buttocks to almost full extension. A rule to note is that the higher the knees are toward the abdomen, the higher the back stretch; conversely, the further away the feet are from the back, the lower the stretch.

Chair Rotation Stretch (Fig. 6-11)

Purpose. To increase a limited trunk rotation.

Space and/or equipment. Straight-back chair.

Starting position. Sit on a chair with hips well back and feet placed firmly on the floor or hooked inside the front legs of the chair. Then rotate the trunk as far around as possible and grasp the back of the chair with both hands. Specifically, the hand of the arm nearest the back of the chair grasps the furthest edge of the chair back while the furthest arm grasps the near edge of the chair back.

Execution
1. Keeping the head and trunk in good alignment, pull the trunk into rotation as much as possible.
2. Repeat one or two times and then change to the opposite direction.

Floor Sitting Trunk Rotation Stretch (Fig. 6-12)

Purpose. To stretch trunk rotators, hip abductors, and front shoulder muscles.

Space and/or equipment. Firm mat.

Starting position. Take a long sitting position. Bend one leg under the other leg. Place the foot of the upper leg over the knee of the bent lower leg. Rotate the trunk as far as possible in the direction of the upper leg. Press the arm that is nearest the hooked upper leg against the knee, with the hand

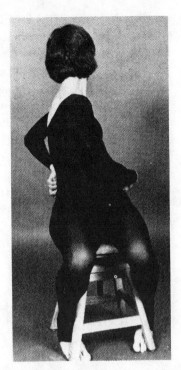

Fig. 6-11. Chair trunk rotation stretch.

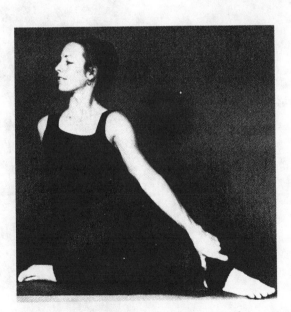

Fig. 6-12. Floor sitting trunk rotation stretch.

grasping the inside of the foot. Then place the free arm as far around the back as possible while placing the hand firmly on the floor.

Execution

1. Sitting up as straight as possible, turn the head toward the support arm while pressing back on the hooked knee with the other arm.
2. Repeat one or two times and then change to the other direction.

Variation. If the position of the stretch is too difficult, modifications can be made. For example, rather than grasping the foot of the hooked leg, grasp the ankle of the bottom leg, or, to make it easier still, keep the bottom leg in a straight position.

Billig Side Wall Stretch (Fig. 6-13)

Purpose. To stretch the hip abductors, primarily the tensor fasciae latae muscle, and to assist in remediation of the problem of the snapping hip.

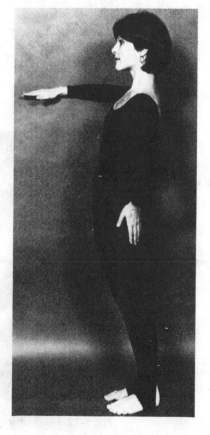

Fig. 6-13. Billig side stretch.

Space and/or equipment. Unobstructed wall.

Starting position. Stand in good postural alignment with feet together and legs straight, one-half an arm's distance from the wall. Place the outside hand in the hollow of the buttocks region while raising the inside arm to shoulder height. Place the forearm against the wall with the elbow slightly forward of the shoulder joint.

Execution

1. Keeping legs and trunk in good alignment, push the pelvis with the outside hand in the direction of the hand positioned on the wall. The pelvis must be maintained at all times at right angles to the wall. The pelvis must not be turned inward.
2. Repeat once and then change to stretch the opposite side.
   CAUTION: Care should be taken not to overly arch the lower back. If pain occurs in the lower back region or there is a history of lower back problems, refrain from performing this stretch.

Fitt Hip Abductor Stretch (Fig. 6-14)

Purpose. To stretch hip abductors, primarily the tensor fasciae latae muscle, and to correct a snapping hip.

Space and/or equipment. Bench or straight-backed chair.

Starting position. With hands placed on the seat of a chair or bench, assume a front resting position with arms straight, supporting the weight of the trunk. Maintain the back and legs in a straight position. Bring the leg forward to a spot approximately in line with the extended leg, and then turn the body so that the hip of the straight leg is facing toward the floor.

Execution

1. Keeping the leg straight at all times, allow the weight of the body to gradually sag directly on the lateral aspect of the hip that is directed toward the floor.
2. Repeat two or three times and then change to stretch the opposite side.
   CAUTION: This stretch may aggravate a knee that has a history of lateral ligament injury and thus should be avoided. Also, this stretch should not be performed if pain is produced in the knee region.

Shoulder Stretch (Fig. 6-15)

Purpose. To stretch both shoulders, with emphasis placed on their anterior aspect.

Space and/or equipment. Mat or stool.

Starting position. While seated either with bent knees or in a cross-legged position on the mat or a stool, raise one arm overhead and backward as far as possible and then bend the elbow and reach down the back as far as possible.

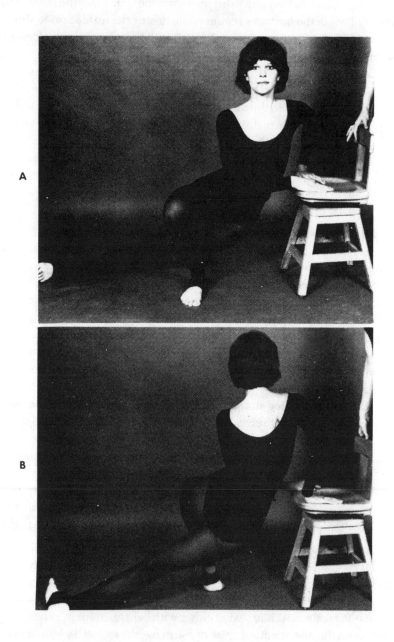

Fig. 6-14. Fitt hip abductor stretch. **A,** Front view. **B,** Back view.

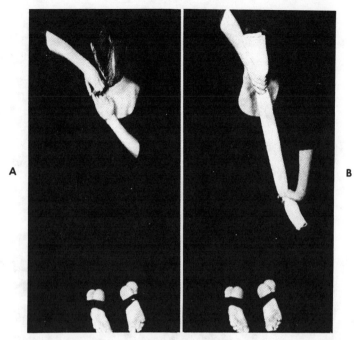

Fig. 6-15. Shoulder stretch. **A,** Grasping fingers. **B,** Using a towel.

With the other arm, reach back as far as possible, bend the elbow, and clasp the other hand.

Execution

1. With the hands clasped, attempt to pull each of the arms closer together.
2. Repeat two or three times and then reverse arm position.

Variation. If unable to clasp the hands, use a towel to pull the shoulders into a stretch.

Key strengthening exercises (Pilates)

Pilates floor work includes a variety of stretch movements directed to the special needs of the dancer. Following are some key Pilates stretches (Fig. 6-16). The exercises presented in this section fall into the category of isotonic (freely moving) or isometric (static) exercises. When isotonic exercise is being performed, the muscle or muscle group becomes shortened; in the case of isometric exercise, the muscle increases in tension and does not become shortened. Exercises that are performed in the full range of joint movement should be conducted in sets of 10 to 15 repetitions with a slow

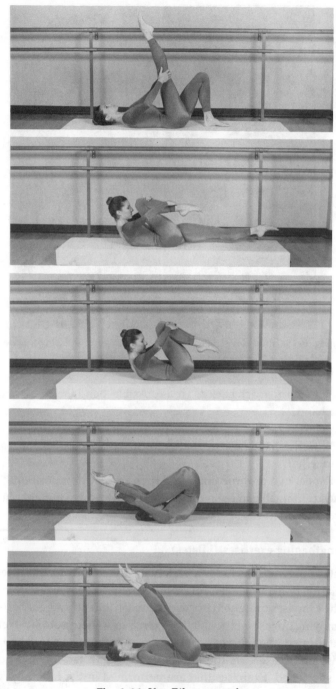

Fig. 6-16. Key Pilates stretches.

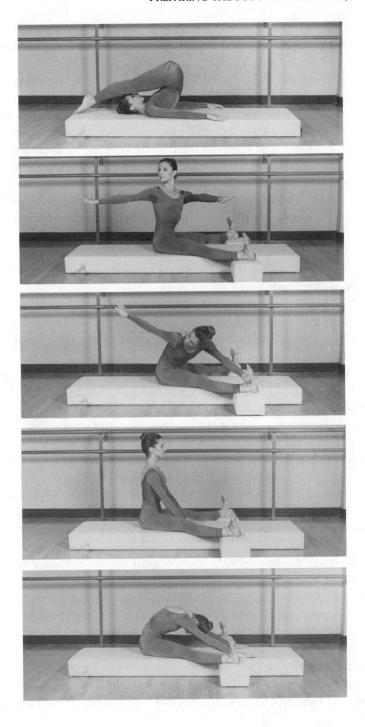

buildup of two or three sets. In contrast, isometric exercises should involve one or two repetitions against an immovable resistance for a maximum of 10 seconds.

Isotonic exercise can be given the added dimension of resistance, especially when greater strength is required than is acquired by free movement against gravity. Resistance can be afforded by a variety of means; for example, weights, self-resistance by one body part resting against another body part, pulleys, rubber tubes, and springs. Overloading a muscle by the application of an external force should be gradual. If the dancer decides to use a weighted object, the DeLorme and Watkins method of overloading is suggested:[10]

1. First, by executing 10 repetitions of a particular movement the dancer should determine the resistance that can be barely overcome. This determines the *maxi bout*.

2. A DeLorme overload routine consists of three sets or bouts of 10 repetitions, with full recovery between each set consisting of about 2 to 5 minutes of rest.

3. The first set of 10 consists of resistance that is equal to one-half that of the maxi bout, the second set consists of resistance equal to three-fourths that of the maxi bout, and the third and last bout consists of a full maxi bout.

4. A good rule of thumb is to add to the resistance when the last set can be performed easily for more than 10 repetitions.

Gathering the Towel (Fig. 6-17)

Purpose. To strengthen the metatarsal and the inner longitudinal arch of the foot and to assist in remediation of the pronated foot.

Space and/or equipment. Bench or chair, towel, and an object to use as a resistance on the end of the towel, such as a book.

Starting position. Sit on the bench or chair with the feet directly under the knees and the heels on the floor. Place the toes on the end of the towel, which has been stretched out in front. Place weighted object on the towel's end.

Execution

1. Keeping the heels firmly planted, pull the towel toward the feet using a scooping action. In the process, keep the toes straight, if possible, performing the scooping action with the ball of the feet. Use each foot alternately until the majority of the towel has been gathered between the feet.

2. Repeat two or three times.

Towel Scoop (Fig. 6-18)

Purpose. To strengthen the inner aspect of the foot and to assist in remediation of the fallen inner longitudinal arch and the pronated foot.

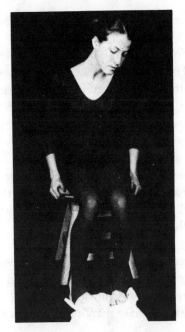

Fig. 6-17. Gathering the towel.

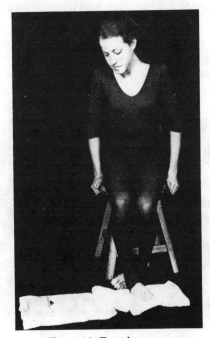

Fig. 6-18. Towel scoop.

Space and/or equipment. Towel, an object for resistance, and a chair or bench.

Starting position. Sit on a chair or bench with the feet directly under the knees and heels placed firmly on the floor. Place the toes of the foot to be exercised at the end of the towel that has been folded in half. The towel is positioned crosswise to the dancer with the object to provide resistance placed on one end. To create a brace, position the opposite foot behind the outside of the heel of the exercising foot.

Execution

1. Keeping the heel firmly fixed on the floor, scoop the towel in a straight line across the front of the legs using the fall of the foot to scoop the towel. Do not try to flex the toes during the exercise.
2. Repeat two or three times.

Foot Lift (Fig. 6-19)

Purpose. To strengthen the muscles that extend the toes and foot backward that are found in the anterior aspect of the lower leg and to possibly assist in the prevention and remediation of shin splints.

Space and/or equipment. Exercise mat or chair and a 2- to 5-pound sandbag.

Starting position. While sitting on a chair or mat, point or extend the foot to be exercised and place the opposite foot directly on top of the extended foot.

Execution

1. With the top foot, apply downward pressure to the exercising foot while attempting to pull it backward. First apply isometric resistance

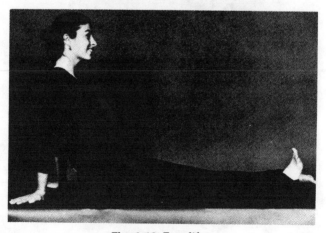

Fig. 6-19. Foot lift.

for 10 seconds, and then pull the foot slowly back through a complete range of motion.

2. Repeat two or three times.

Knee Rotator (Fig. 6-20)

Purpose. To assist in the remediation of knock-knees, tibial torsion, pronated feet, and fallen longitudinal arch.

Space and/or equipment. Barre or a straight-backed chair.

Starting position. While holding on to a barre or the back of a straight-backed chair with both hands, stand with heels 3 inches apart, big toes touching each other, and weight borne on the outside of each foot.

Execution

1. While flexing the knees slightly, rotate the knees vigorously outward, causing the heels to resist being forced inward. If this is performed correctly, a high longitudinal arch will form and a high degree of muscle tension will be felt on the outsides of the knees.

2. Perform each rotation for 10 seconds and repeat two or three times.

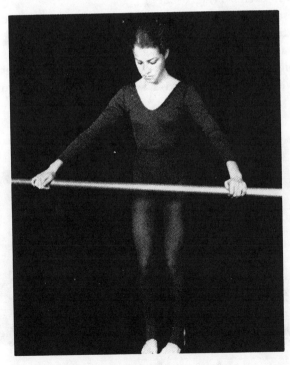

Fig. 6-20. Knee rotator.

Hip Abduction with Internal Rotation (Fig. 6-21)

Purpose. To strengthen the hip abductors, specifically the gluteus medium muscle, and to offset the fact that dancers typically have weak hip abductors and overly strong external rotators. Characteristically, a dancer performs a battement tendu, a grand battement, or like movements that utilize those muslces that bring the hip into flexion and external rotation rather than into abduction. Also, to assist in the remediation of a snapping hip.

Space and/or equipment. Exercise mat and a weight to be fixed to the ankle.

Starting position. Assume a side-lying position with legs straight and feet together.

Execution

1. With the leg internally rotated, abduct the hip through a full range of movement.
2. Perform in sets of 10 repetitions and work to a maximum of three sets.

Variation. Rather than side-lying, stand and perform the same exercise. Add a weight to the ankle for resistance, starting with 2 pounds.

Bring-to Exercise (Fig. 6-22)

Purpose. To strengthen the hip adductors and to assist in the prevention and remediation of groin strain.

Space and/or equipment. Exercise mat.

Starting position. Assume a side-lying position with both legs straight and the upper leg positioned from 12 to 18 inches above the bottom leg.

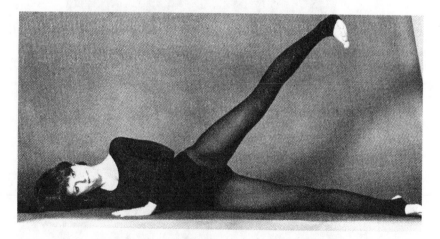

Fig. 6-21. Hip abduction with internal rotation.

Execution

1. Lift the bottom leg to meet the upper leg. When both legs are together off of the floor, hold this position for 10 seconds. Then slowly return the bottom leg to the mat.
2. Repeat two or three times and change to exercise the other leg.

Variation. While sitting or reclining, spread and bring both legs together, sliding them on the floor.

Leg Weight Series (Fig. 6-23)

Many free leg exercises can be assisted with leg weights weighing 2- to 5-pounds placed around the ankle. This added stress can provide increased strength and endurance. Each exercise should be repeated up to 10 repetitions in one to three sets of 10.

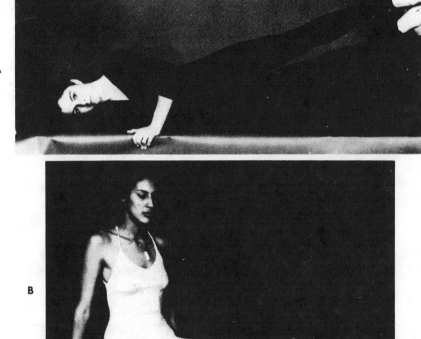

Fig. 6-22. A, Hip adduction with the lower leg raised to meet the abducted upper leg. **B,** Hip adduction while seated.

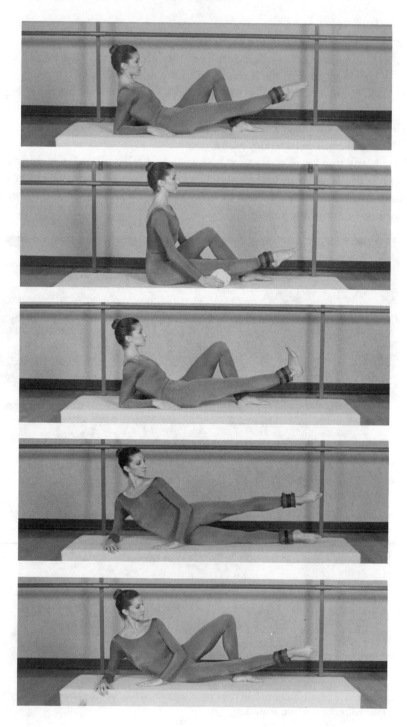

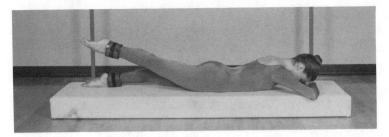

Fig. 6-23. Left and above. Leg weight series.

Leg Circles (Fig. 6-24)

Purpose. To stabilize hip and increase its range of motion.

Space and/or equipment. Back-lying position, leg extended with hip at 90 degrees flexion, toes pointed.

Execution

1. With the leg at right angles to the body perform 10 internal hip rotations and 10 external rotations. Repeat two to three times.
2. With the leg abducted repeat #1 sequence.
3. With the leg adducted repeat #1 sequence.

Knee and Elbow Touch (Fig. 6-25)

Purpose. To strengthen the abdominal muscles.

Space and/or equipment. Exercise mat.

Starting position. Lie on the back with knees in a hooklike position and hands clasped behind the neck.

Execution

1. While curling the head forward, touch one elbow to the tip of the opposite knee and return slowly to the mat; then repeat with the opposite elbow and knee.
2. Repeat up to three sets of 10 repetitions each.

Abdominal Curl (Fig. 6-26)

Purpose. To strengthen the abdominal muscles.

Space and/or equipment. Exercise mat.

Starting position. Assume a hook-lying position, with hands clasped behind the head, and curl the trunk upward.

Execution

1. While curling the head forward and touching the chin to the chest, slowly curl up and touch the elbows to the knees and then slowly return to the starting postion.
2. Repeat one to three sets of 10 repetitions per set.

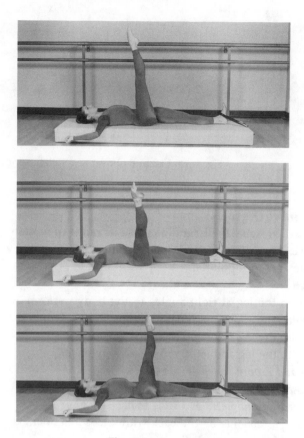

Fig. 6-24. Leg circles.

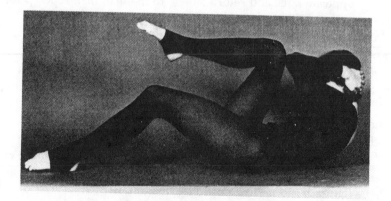

Fig. 6-25. Knee and elbow touch.

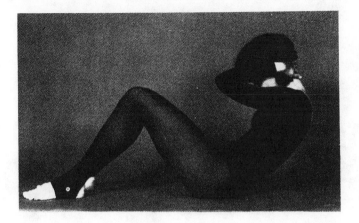

Fig. 6-26. Abdominal curl.

Mad Cat (Fig. 6-27)

Purpose. To strengthen abdominal, shoulder, and back muscles and to assist in the remediation of lumbar lordosis and inflexible lower back.

Space and/or equipment. Exercise mat.

Starting position. Assume a four-point kneeling position while keeping the head in line with the trunk and the back straight. Place the hands directly under the shoulders.

Execution

    1. Drop the head down, hump the back, and suck in the abdominal muscles as far as possible. While holding this position, bend the elbows and touch the forehead to the mat just in front of the fingertips. Keeping the back humped, return to the four-point position, lift the head, and straighten the back.

    2. Repeat two or three times.

Side Lift (Fig. 6-28)

Purpose. To strengthen the lateral trunk flexors and to assist in the remediation of scoliosis and/or lateral hip tilt.

Space and/or equipment. Exercise mat.

Starting position. Assume a side-lying position with legs straight and feet together. While resting on one forearm, extend the other arm to shoulder height.

Execution

    1. Raise the hips sideways off the mat as far as possible and hold that position for 10 seconds.

    2. Repeat two or three times and then change to the other side.

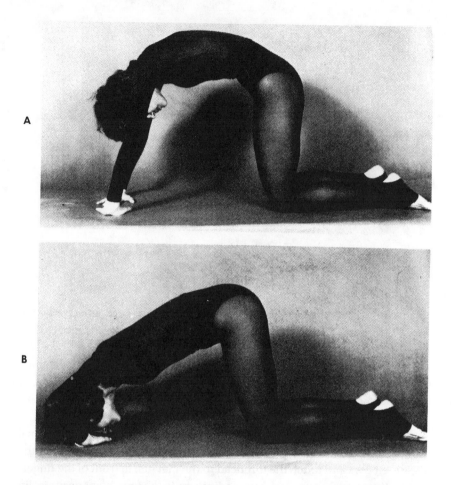

Fig. 6-27. Mad cat. **A,** Rounding the back. **B,** While attempting to hold the back rounded, the dancer lowers her head to the mat and then pushes up to a straight arm position.

CAUTION: If the exercise is used to correct "C"-type scoliosis, the convexity of the curve should be positioned toward the mat.

Chest and Arm Raise (Fig. 6-29)

Purpose. To strengthen the extensor muscles of the back and neck and to assist in the remediation of round back, kyphosis, and winged scapula.

Space and/or equipment. Exercise mat.

Starting position. Lie face down.

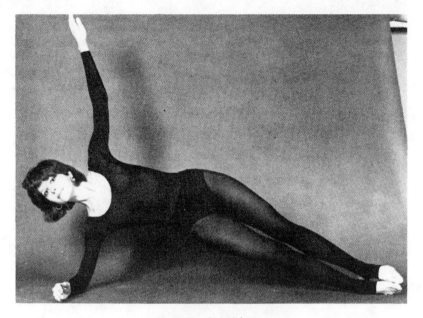

Fig. 6-28. Side lift.

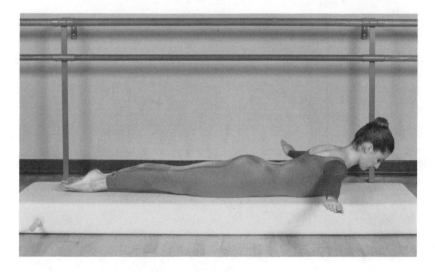

Fig. 6-29. Chest and arm raise.

Execution

1. Raise the head so that the face, neck, and upper chest are off the mat, and at the same time bring the arms out to the side, pinching the scapula together. Hold this position for 10 seconds.
2. Repeat two or three times.

   CAUTION: The dancer should keep the abdomen and pelvis in contact with the mat and avoid arching the lower back.

7

Nutrition

When the dancer considers all the factors that help to prevent bodily injury as well as those that assist in healing the body when injury does occur, nutrition must be considered as one of the most important. Because of the demands of dance, what is ingested into the body must be of the highest quality and appropriate to the individual needs of the performer.[26] The dancer tends toward food fallacies and fadism that often serve to hamper performance and even delay the healing process.[6]

This chapter is devoted to presenting the most current information on sensible nutritional practices for the individual who engages in a high level of physical activity. Most professional dancers fail to eat correctly and are deficient in the basic nutrients.

NUTRITIONAL GUIDELINES

In order for dancers to engage in strenuous activities, their bodies must have sufficient nutrients to properly supply the working muscles. Good nutrition involves the daily intake of four primary food groups in balanced amounts to provide normal organic function. These groups are: milk and milk products; meat, fish, poultry, and alternatives; breads and cereals; and fruits and vegetables. Each must be ingested into the body in certain amounts. For energy, carbohydrates should constitute 55% or more of the diet, fat from 25% to 30% (only being saturated fats), and proteins from 10% to 12%, together with proper amounts of vitamins, minerals, and water.

Carbohydrates

Carbohydrates, which are made up of the elements of carbon, hydrogen, and oxygen, are found in such food substances as starches, sugars, bread stuffs, potatoes, and rice. When ingested into the body they become readily available as energy sources. Carbohydrates are stored in the liver as glycogen and serve to overcome the sense of fatigue when there is a sugar depletion in the blood.

Fats

Fat, although similar in composition to carbohydrates, is present in a more complex form. Fats are usually stored in the body as a reserve source of fuel as energy. Because of the difficulty of utilization, fat is not considered as ready a source of energy as carbohydrates.

Protein

Protein is mainly used by the body for tissue building, repair of tissue, and regulation of body functions. Contrary to current thought among many dancers, more than 10% to 12% of protein in the diet does not add markedly to strength or endurance. Only in an extremely heavy strength overload program does the body use the greater percentage of protein.

Vitamins

The organic compounds known as vitamins do not function as energy producers nor do they build tissue, although they do catalyze other organic compounds to produce energy and build tissue. At this time, approximately 26 vitamins have been identified. Of these, vitamins A, B complex, and D are the most well known. Vitamin A is essential for cellular growth and assists in combating bacterial infection; deficiency in vitamin A produces night blindness. Vitamin A is found in red or orange foods, such as carrots, and in leafy vegetables. Vitamin B complex (B_1, B_2, and B_{12}) is essential for the function of enzymes, utilization of carbohydrates, normal growth, and basic organic functions. Because vitamin B complex has a water base, it is not stored in the body and must be taken in the diet on a daily basis. It can be found in liver, brewer's yeast, fruits, and vegetables. Vitamin C is probably the most unstable of all vitamins and is also water soluble. Vitamin C is essential for the formation of the material that binds cells together. It is essential in the healing of injuries such as often occur to soft tissue. It also assists the dancer in combating stress. Vitamin C is found in citrus fruits and many vegetables, such as cabbage. Vitamin D, like vitamin A, has an oil base and is stored in the body. An overdose of either one of these vitamins may be toxic. Vitamin D is essential for bone growth and cellular function. It is found commonly in milk, cod liver oil, and fish.

Minerals

Of all the nutritional substances, minerals are probably the least understood. However, as a common food element they are essential for the proper functioning of the body and for the maintenance of life. Without the proper balance of such minerals as calcium, sodium, potassium, and magnesium, normal cellular function is possible. Other trace elements such as cobalt, copper, iodine, manganese, and iron are essential for various cellular functions. The physically active person will experience many symptoms stemming from decreased amounts of minerals in the body, such as muscle cramping, fatigue, and slow recovery from the effects of physical activity. A balanced diet, which contains an abundance of water and a variety of vegetables, should provide the mineral requirements of the body.

If the dancer takes in the basic food groups in the correct proportions each day, the nutrients required for a vigorous and physically active life will be provided. The major foods necessary for efficient physical activity are milk, meats, vegetables and fruits, and breads and cereals. The dancer should avoid food fads and strive for a balanced approach to eating (Table 2).

Water

Adequate intake of water is essential to the dancer's health. Water makes up 75% of all protoplasm. It acts as a dilutent for toxic wastes, transports body fuels, eliminates waste materials, and regulates body temperature.

Dehydration must not be allowed to happen; a lack of water depletes the body of minerals and may cause cramping, leading to muscle tears. Sixteen ounces of water should be ingested about a half-an-hour before performing and 6 ounces ingested every 15 minutes in conditions of heat and/or humidity. The dancer must remember the sensation of thirst is not a good indicator of the body's need for water. A 2% to 3% body weight loss through perspiration may be cause for concern, especially if it is not replaced by the next day.

FOOD SUPPLEMENTATION

A current tendency among physically active people, particularly those individuals who are continuously dieting, is to supplement their diets with vitamin and protein pills. For the most part, unless there is a deficiency, this practice does little good and is probably a waste of money. A balanced diet will provide all that an active person requires. However, the individual who eats irregularly and realizes that his or her diet is not complete should take

Table 2. Food Guide to Healthy Eating (Avoids Fat, Sugar, and Salt)*

1. **Milk and Milk Products**

    Children up to 11 years   2—3 servings
    Adolescents   3—4 servings
    Adults   2 servings
    One serving is:
    1 cup of milk, ¾ cup yogurt, 1½ ounces cheddar or processed cheese

2. **Meat, Fish, Poultry and Alternatives**

    3-4 servings per day
    One serving is:
    2—3 ounces cooked lean meat, fish, poultry or liver
    4 tablespoons peanut butter
    1 cup cooked dried peas, beans or lentils
    ½ cup nuts or seeds
    2 ounces cheddar cheese
    ½ cup cottage cheese
    2 eggs

3. **Breads and Cereals**

    3—5 servings per day (whole grain foods are recommended)
    One serving is:
    1 slice bread
    ½ cup cooked cereal
    ¾ cup ready-to-eat cereal
    1 roll or muffin
    ½—¾ cup cooked rice, macaroni, spaghetti, or noodles
    ½ hamburger or wiener bun

4. **Fruits and Vegetables**

    4-5 servings per day (include at least two vegetables). Choose a variety of both vegetables
    and fruits—include yellow, green, and green leafy vegetables.
    One serving is:
    ½ cup vegetables or fruit (fresh, frozen, or canned)
    ½ cup juice
    1 medium-sized potato, carrot, tomato, peach, apple, orange, or banana

*Adapted from Canada's Food Guide, *Health and Welfare*, Canada, 1983.

supplements containing the minimum daily requirements of vitamins and minerals. High-potency vitamins should be avoided, especially potentially toxic vitamins such as A and D. Increasing vitamin dosage in an unscientific manner may disrupt the delicate organic chemical balance of the body.

FOOD ROUTINES

Dancers are concerned about what types of food to consume before a performance. In actuality, pre-dance performance nutrition must vary with the dancer. However, research does indicate that gastric distress due to nervousness can be alleviated to a great extent if a meal is eaten approximately 3 hours before a performance. This allows the food to be digested out of the stomach and into the intestinal tract. This is not to say, however, that the dancer should go into a performance hungry; hunger may adversely affect performance. It is suggested that those who feel hunger pangs before performing should drink a 4- to 6-ounce can of liquid diet drink. Intake of a diet drink will statiate hunger pangs and at the same time provide some bulk for the stomach without causing distress or gas. The foods that can be eaten during the period before performance should be those that are high in complex carbohydrates. Animal fat and protein, as well as foods containing sugar should be avoided. In other words, it is suggested that foods be selected from those that are easily digested (Table 3).

A dancer who sits down to a meal 4 hours before a vigorous performance has most of the food out of the stomach before activity commences.

Table 3. Approximate time required for foods to leave the stomach

beef, 3 hours;
lamb or pork, 3¼ hours;
vegetables and fruits, 2¾ hours;
desserts such as cake, 3½ hours;
cereal products, 2½ hours;
milk, 2¾ hours

WEIGHT CONTROL

Weight control is one of the most difficult problems the dancer has to face. Eating habits, individual absorption rates, and individual food idiosyncrasies play an important role in whether the dancer maintains the correct body weight. The problem of losing weight often causes the dancer to engage in fads and harmful diet practices that result in less than optimum functioning of the entire body. Because of an overconcern for thinness, some dancers engage in the gorge/purge cycle known as bulimia or develop the psychological condition known as *anorexia nervosa*, which leads to a loss of appetite and subsequent loss of body weight, possibly leading to death (Table 4).

Table 4. Recognizing the Athlete with an Eating Disorder*

Signs to look for are dancers who display

1. Social isolation and withdrawal from friends and family
2. A lack of confidence in dance abilities
3. Ritualistic eating behavior (e.g., organizing food on plate)
4. An obsession with counting calories
5. An obsession with constantly exercising, especially just before a meal
6. An obsession with weighing self
7. A constant overestimation of body size
8. Patterns of leaving the table directly after eating to go into the restroom
9. Problems related to eating disorders (e.g., malnutrition, menstrual irregularities, or chronic fatigue)

*Adapted from Arnheim, D.D.: Modern principles of athletic training, ed. 7, St. Louis: Times Mirror/Mosby College Publishing, 1989.

Bulimia is considered a neurotic eating disorder that is common among dancers.[6] It is characterized by bouts of overeating followed by voluntary vomiting, fasting, and use of laxatives or diuretics. Typically the bulimics gorge themselves with high-caloried food after a period of starvation and then "purge" themselves. Such behavior disrupts heart rhythm, and causes stomach rupture and liver damage. Vomiting, which brings up stomach acids, can decay teeth and inflame the mucous lining of the mouth and throat.[8] It can also cause amenorrhea.[9]

The dancer must practice an intelligent approach to weight control, avoiding fads and eating a balanced diet and should not be allowed to dance below a healthy weight.

Simply said, excess weight is caused by taking in more energy in food than the body expends in activity. To lose weight the dancer must reverse this process. However, rapid weight loss in a short period may be harmful; therefore, every effort must be expended to lose weight over a long period. No more than 2 or 3 pounds should be lost in a week. Fat that is taken off gradually has a tendency to stay off, whereas weight that is lost rapidly tends to be replaced rapidly. The crash diet serves only to increase susceptibility to diseases resulting from low resistance. Crash diets can also lead to chronic fatigue and susceptibility to traumatic injuries.

The best way to acheive weight reduction is to eat a balanced diet but decrease the number of calories ingested during the day. If the dancer who has a normal metabolism decreases the normal daily calorie intake by 500 calories, ½ pound of fat can be lost about every 3 days.

Because of variations in body build, particularly among female dancers, many desire to spot reduce certain areas of the body such as the hips and thighs. Research has shown that spot reduction is extremely unlikely by the sweat method. The practice of wearing special plastic or rubberized spot reduction garments that are localized to one area are of little value. In fact, there may even be some danger in wearing plastic sweat suits that do not allow the body to ventilate properly. The best means of spot reduction is by an exercise program involving many repetitions in a full range of movement and involving numerous muscle contractions in the specific area; for example, for reducing the hips, the dancer lies on one side and executes 20 to 30 leg lifts, bringing the side of the leg as high as possible and down. This method discourages heavy muscle development and encourages longer muscle fibers to develop, as well as reducing the amount of fat in the area.

Weight gain, on the other hand, is best attained by increasing the amount of food intake beyond the daily expenditure. However, the intake of an overabundance of fatty foods should be discouraged.

The method of using height and weight charts for determining optimum body weight must be considered inaccurate and too general for the dancer to follow. The best means of determining the amount of fat distribution in the body is by use of skinfold calipers. The most characteristic fat area for both men and women is the triceps area (back of arm). Other areas of fat accumulation are the abdominal area, the buttocks, and the suprailiac and subscapular regions. Because dancers appear heavier on stage, on television, and in movies, skinfold measurements at these sites should probably not exceed 8 to 10 mm for adult females and 6 to 8 mm for adult males. In terms of total body fat, it is desirable for the male, in general, not to exceed 13% to 15% total body fat and the female, 15% to 25%.

The safest way for dancers to control their food consumption and thus maintain the proper weight is to become acutely aware of their own intake and energy output. To do this the dancer should make a carefully noted 2-week diary of all food taken into the body. This means measures of sugar, weights of meat, ounces of beverages, etc. Once the amount of the week's food has been accumulated, the calories of the specific foods should be determined by using a simple calorie counter that can be purchased from any grocery store. This week's intake is added and then divided by 7 to provide the average daily calorie intake. During the same week that the dancer develops a food intake diary, a diary of the amount and intensity of physical activity should also be kept. Using Table 5, the dancer can estimate how many calories he or she expends in one 24-hour period. The dancer then knows, based on the amount of activity engaged in, how many average calories per day are maintaining the dancer at a particular weight level. If weight loss is desired, the practice of decreasing the average daily calorie intake by 500 calories should provide a safe 2-pound weight reduction per week and

Table 5. Calculation of daily energy requirement*

Activity level	Calories/lb/hr
Sleeping	0.43
Sitting (watching TV, eating, etc.)	0.67
Light exercise (social dancing, tennis, jogging, dance practice, etc.)	1.95
Severe exercise (dance performance, competitive sports such as racquetball, etc.)	3.00

Determine the amount of time that each activity level is engaged in by multiplying the constant on the right side of the chart times your body weight to give the amount of calories per pound per hour.

NOTE: Be careful not to overestimate the amount of time spent in an activity, especially severe exercise.

*Modified from Crowe, W.C., Arnheim, D.D., and Auxter, D.: Laboratory manual in adapted physical education and recreation; experiments, activities, and assignments, St. Louis: The C.V. Mosby Co., 1977.

conversely, increasing the intake by 500 calories should add about 2 to 3 pounds per week. It is important to note that any diet to control weight must have a daily balance of the basic four food groups.

Another method of losing weight is by decreasing the number of servings in the basic four food groups (Table 6).

Table 6. Basic Four Food Groups Diet Allowance

Food group	Servings
Milk	One cup of milk or equivalent
Fruits and vegetables	One serving of green or yellow vegetables One serving of citrus fruit, tomato, or cabbage Two or more servings of other fruits and vegetables, including potato
Breads and cereals	Three servings of whole-grain or enriched cereals or breads
Protein-rich foods	One serving of egg, meat, fish, poultry, cheese, dried beans, or peas One or more additional servings of egg, meat, fish, poultry, or cheese

Crash Dieting

Dancers often "crash" diet. This practice can be dangerous to the dancer's health. It causes a lowering of energy level and can lead to colds and infections.

This in turn can lead to a serious injury. As stated earlier, the only safe way to diet is to reduce caloric intake or servings of the basic food groups.[3]

HEAT STRESS

The dancer's reaction to high temperatures is very important. Hot stage lights and poor air circulation can contribute to extreme temperatures and cause serious physiological problems for the dancer. Often adding to these heat conditions are costumes that keep heat in, not allowing perspiration to evaporate and cool the body. The dancer can lose from 2 to 6 pounds of water in one performance. When the temperature exceeds 89°F, the only means by which the body can dissipate heat is through perspiration. If the humidity is also high, evaporation is restricted and sweating may not adequately cool the body, causing the internal temperature of the dancer to rise. The first indication of adverse effects of heat are muscle cramps that result from excess perspiration and the elimination of salt and other minerals from the body. Excessive mineral loss increases motor nerve excitability and results in cramping. When the dancer continues to work on cramped muscles, the results are muscle pulls and perhaps even tears. If a dancer insists on continuing to dance while experiencing high temperatures and humidity, heat exhaustion can occur.

Heat exhaustion is caused by a depletion of body fluids and results in a general letdown of the body processes such as commonly seen in shock. The dancer complains of extreme fatigue and chills and has cold beads of sweat on the forehead, under the eyes, and on the upper lip. The pulse is rapid and weak. Under such circumstances, the dancer should be treated symtomatically. If there is a sense of coldness, the dancer should be covered and, of course, taken out of the adverse environment and allowed to rest. If the dancer continues to exercise while experiencing heat exhaustion, a very serious complication known as heat stroke could arise.

Heat stroke presents a different set of symptoms than those of heat exhaustion. The dancer may collapse, the skin is dry, the heart rate is very slow and weak, the face may be red, and breathing comes in labored gasps. Under these circumstances, immediate medical attention must be sought. The dancer must be cooled down immediately, because the internal body temperature may reach as high as 106°F and death could follow. Immediate care should include removing tight clothing and placing cold, wet cloths on the back of the neck, the stomach, the legs, and under the arms, followed by rapid fanning to drop the temperature as quickly as possible. If ice is available, it is preferable to cold, wet cloths.

Most individuals can become acclimatized to extremely adverse environmental conditions, including high temperatures and humidity; however, acclimatization takes from 1 to 2 weeks. Under adverse climatic conditions, the dancer should practice during the coolest time of day and in the beginning should not work more than half an hour at a time. Fluid should be taken when needed, and the dancer should be cognizant of the amount of weight loss that occurs following each practice session. It has been determined that 2% to 3% or more weight loss due to perspiration during one exercise period demands special concern. As discussed earlier fluid replacement is extremely important. A final precaution is that the dancer should not attempt weight reduction in adversely hot climatic conditions.

QUESTIONABLE PRACTICES FOR INCREASING ENERGY

The term *ergogenic* means work-producing and is used in the context of physical activity to describe agents taken into the body for the express purpose of improving performance. Besides substances taken into the system, an ergogen can also be a motivational technique designed to improve performance. In today's society it is becoming commonplace to take various substances to increase performance or to delay the onset of the feeling of fatigue. Some dancers attempt to improve their performance by questionable practices. These include the use of stimulants such as coffee and tea, or even amphetamines, such as Benzedrine or Dexedrine. Amphetamines (pep pills) function as powerful stimulants to the central nervous system, which increase the heart rate and blood pressure and produce a general feeling of alertness and well-being. Amphetamines are used by people engaged in physical activity most often to overcome the feeling of fatigue. Some individuals react adversely to amphetamines, which may produce dizziness, depression, hallucinations, and poor judgment. Users of pep pills often believe a performance is going well when in actuality it is mediocre or even poor.

Sugar is a substance that, if properly used, can improve endurance. Table sugar, dextrose, glucose, and honey may eventually provide energy for muscle contraction. However, nutritionists indicate that the ingestion of these substances has little effect on activities of short duration. In cases where prolonged muscular contraction is to be engaged in, as in a dance class or performance, the practice of ingesting increased amounts of sugar may be beneficial. In reality, sugar taken orally by itself tends to draw fluid from the body into the gastrointestinal tract and somewhat dehydrates the individual, and sugared drinks tend to reduce the speed with which the fluid is removed from the stomach.

8

Psychological factors
in dance injuries

The psychological aspect of injury prevention is as important to the dancer as is proper conditioning and nutrition. Dancers, like all people, have varying personalities and react to stress in unique ways. What sets dancers off as unique from other individuals is that they are artists seeking perfection in movement. The dancer can have peculiarities that may enhance or detract from the desired neuromuscular control. No artistic endeavor places the mental and emotional demands on the individual that dance does. Consequently, psychological and emotional maturity is as important to the dancer as physical conditioning. The extent to which the dancer can withstand the pyschological stresses imposed by the dance environment is determined by the dancer's total psychoemotional development and lifestyle, both past and present.

ACCIDENT-PRONENESS

The accident-prone dancer is one who experiences more injuries than would be considered normal. In general, there are two times at which accidents normally have a higher incidence: at the beginning of a new series of dance classes or a new production and at the end of a series of classes or a production. One can speculate that the increased number of injuries at the beginning may be due to the dancer's attempts to execute techniques beyond the present ability level or due to inadequate conditioning. At the end of a particular set of classes, injuries may be due to fatigue, both mental and physical, in which the dancer fails to listen to what the body is saying and to avoid dangerous situations.

In the dance field, as in other highly intense physical endeavors, three types of physiological accident-proneness seem to stand out: actually being injured, imagining an injury, and faking an injury.

The accident-prone dancer who is actually injured may be characterized by the fact that the injuries can be identified by the presence of specific pathological conditions. It can be speculated that the cause of the actually-injured type may be a subconscious desire for punishment. The dancer may work to the point that the body actually breaks down or may continually place the body in dangerous situations in which injury is imminent.

On the other hand, individuals whose injuries are imagined are those who feel pain but in whom close medical scrutiny reveals no pathological condition. These individuals are much like a fine clock wound too tightly. They set their sights too high and are unable to attain their aspirations; consequently, they escape through imagined injury. Imagined injuries are often seen in dancers just before participating in a new work or just before going on stage. This reaction to fear is normal. However, it is the individual who year after year has imagined injuries that detract from his or her normal functioning that can be considered psychologically unsound. All people who expose themselves in some way to public scrutiny normally get butterflies in their stomach, their heart speeds up, and they sweat before "going on"; however, the psychologically impaired individual may not be able to "go on" and perhaps escapes the unpleasant feeling through an imagined injury.

The malingerer, on the other hand, is the individual who purposely falsifies an injury to escape work or a personally uncomfortable situation. This individual must be classified as psychologically immature and unable to face life's problems in an adult manner and must be dealt with firmly.

It is not the intent of this text to discuss in detail the psychological factors that make up the complex matrix of human behavior. However, it is important to provide the reader with these more apparent psychological factors that make a dancer more or less prone to injury. It is always good to understand why a dancer chooses dance as a field for self-expression. Understanding why dancers dance can also give an indication of why one dancer is accident-prone while another is seldom bothered by any physical disturbance.

MUSCULAR TENSION AND DANCE

When considering injuries associated with psychogenic factors, one must consider muscular tension as a major cause in the dance field. Tension is defined as increased muscular contraction as a result of some emotional state or muscular work. Nervous tension is a syndrome that is characteristic of the so-called fast way of life of our times. It is associated with anxiety that comes from an undefined worry or fear. An overanxious dancer can have an extremely high level of unneeded muscular tension. The person who is outwardly anxious may be less flexible and less able to smoothly coordinate muscles. Organically he or she may have an increased heart rate and blood pressure. The tense dancer is extremely susceptible to injury and because of this increased muscular excitability may overrespond to painful conditions. The ability to eliminate muscular tension by consciously "letting go" is very important to all dancers. Dancers who can relax at will can increase their mental and physical efficiency.

Respiration, circulation, and coordination are positively affected when relaxation is controlled. For example, there is a more efficient exchange of oxygen and carbon dioxide when the muscles of inspiration and expiration are without tension. Blood can circulate unimpeded when the blood vessels are not overly constricted by the pressure of the musculature, and the dancer is more easily able to engage in differential relaxation, which allows smooth coordination of the agonist and antagonist muscles.

Although anxiety must be controlled when the dancer is engaged in activity over a long period, preperformance jitters or tension is considered normal. Even the most experienced dancer goes through this syndrome, sometimes to the point of nausea and vomiting. However, once on stage the professional soon forgets the fear and performs effectively. The preperformance jitters are nature's way of preparing the dancer for maximal expenditure of energy. The primary glands that bring about the readiness state are the adrenal glands, which secrete the hormone adrenalin as part of their function. Adrenalin is released into the bloodstream to speed up circulation and respiration and to assist in bringing fuel to the muscles. It also increases the removal of metabolites and other waste products from the muscles. Associated with the readiness state may be feelings of anxiety, breathlessness, butterflies in the stomach to the point of nausea, dry mouth, and an increase in the action of the bowels. All of these are normal responses to getting ready to perform. Without this reaction to the forthcoming performance, the dancer may in fact be put in a situation where an injury might be incurred. The readiness condition places the body in a state that makes injury less likely.

STALENESS

Staleness is a period of physical and emotional letdown that usually follows a long period of intense physical exertion and is associated with an inability to relax and rest comfortably. It may also be associated with a loss of appetite, digestive problems, weight loss, and a general feeling of lethary (Table 7). Staleness is common among dancers during periods when there has been an extremely long session of practice without letup or after a very discouraging tour in which expectations have not been met. In such cases the dancer feels fatigue and extreme letdown with an inability to get emotionally "up" for the next performance.

Table 7. Recognizing signs of staleness in dancers

The dancer who is becoming stale may display some of the following signs. He or she may:

1. Display a decrease in performance level
2. Have difficulty falling asleep
3. Be awakened from sleep for no apparent reason
4. Experience a loss of weight or, conversely, overeat
5. Have indigestion
6. Have difficulty concentrating
7. Have difficulty enjoying sex
8. Have nausea for no apparent reason
9. Be prone to head colds and/or allergic reactions
10. Act restless, irritable, anxious, and/or depressed
11. Have an elevated resting heart rate and blood pressure
12. Show psychomatic episodes

Because staleness is primarily a mental state rather than a physical problem, it is best handled by reasoning or by a change of pace. When staleness is apparent, the dancer should completely change his or her environment and do something entirely different. If this is not possible, the dancer should at least attempt to change the pace by varying a basic routine. Sometimes just a little praise from an important person can make all the difference in the world to a dancer who is becoming stale. The dancer who is in a stale period is extremely susceptible to injury, and injury situations must be avoided at all cost. Accident-proneness is very probable during this emotionally low period.

IV

PRINCIPLES OF INJURY CARE

Part IV provides important information to intelligently evaluate injuries arising from dance. It also gives a commonsense rationale for applying immediate and follow-up care for the most prevalent conditions occurring in dance.

9

Evaluating physical trauma in dance

Everyone associated with the dance profession should be able to recognize and intelligently evaluate the seriousness of injuries stemming from dancing. Too often, because of time schedules, ignorance, or carelessness, dance injuries are neglected to the extent that they cause unnecessary pain, disability, and loss of time.

Because dancers may often exceed the limits of their bodies or inadvertently place themselves in situations where violent forces are imposed, the body becomes traumatized. Traumatic injuries may be categorized as either internal or external. External injuries are the exposed type and include such skin conditions as blisters, abrasions (scrapes), lacerations (tears), and incisions (cuts). Internal injuries are for the most part unexposed, constituting conditions of the musculoskeletal system such as contusions, strains, sprains, dislocations, and fractures as well as injury to the internal organs of the body in some cases.

INFLAMMATION AND HEALING

The inflammatory process is involved in both exposed and unexposed injuries. Inflammation occurs when body tissues are irritated and react with redness, heat, swelling, pain, and in some cases cellular malfunctioning. Whatever the irritant may be—traumatic, chemical, thermal, or pathogenic— cellular disruption results in metabolic changes that produce inflammation, which in general, is a protective process designed to repair and heal the body.

When an injury occurs, a vascular reaction brings about a fluid imbalance at the injury site. At the moment trauma occurs, blood vessels and capillaries constrict at the point of tissue insult, emptying the area of blood for a short period. Following constriction, capillary dilation occurs, which allows a flood of blood and serum into the area of injury. This fluid causes pressure on exposed nerve endings, resulting in pain. At the time of tissue insult, hormones direct white blood cells to the area to begin the process of removing debris from the area. At the same time, repair and healing begin, as the injured site becomes organized into a blood clot that later becomes a fibrous scar.

Ideally, healing should take place with as little scarring as possible. Scar tissue basically is an inferior tissue and is susceptible to repeated injuries. Two types of injury healing occur: primary healing, or healing by first intention, and secondary healing, or healing by second intention. Primary healing is the type of healing that produces little scarring because the edges of the wound are closely approximated. Secondary healing is the type of healing that occurs where there has been a great deal of tissue damage, and the edges of the wound are gapped. Most traumatic injuries of the body heal by secondary intention. Injuries that are given proper immediate care and not allowed to become chronic will develop a minimum of scar tissue.

ACUTE INJURIES

Dancers are susceptible to acute musculoskeletal problems caused by forces that overly stretch or compress selected tissues of the body. A force that causes a sudden insult to the body produces an acute injury that, if managed properly, should be of short duration.

Four procedures are usually followed in the initial stages of caring for an acute injury to assist nature in the inflammation process and repair. These four procedures are compression, cold, elevation, and proper rest. Compression of the injury helps prevent the accumulation of fluids; cold applied to an area constricts superficial blood vessels and helps keep fluid accumulation (edema) and swelling under control; elevation slows the circulation at the injured site; and rest allows the body to effectively carry on the healing process. Immediate care properly applied does not reduce the pathological damage actually present in the area, but compression, cold, elevation, and rest help make the injured area more amenable to follow-up.

Contusion. There is a high incidence of contusions, or acute compressions, to the bodies of active people. A contusion is a bruise resulting in variable degrees of pathological damage, depending on the force of the blow and its body locality. A contusion can crush tissue, disrupting the continuity of capillaries, and cause swelling or occasionally result in a hematoma, or blood tumor. A hematoma can be described as the localization of the bleeding site into a clot surrounded by a connective tissue membrane. A severe contusion can cause extreme pain, swelling, and in some cases a temporary paralysis caused by the combined pressure of the swelling and muscle spasm on nerves.

Muscle strain. Muscle strain, which is caused by an overstretching of the musculotendinous unit (the entire muscle and the tendons), is the most common problem that the dancer must face. It can range from a mild stretch to a complete rupture or avulsion (tearing of the tendinous tissue away from its place of insertion). The exact cause of muscle strain is often very difficult to ascertain but often is due to a breakdown in the reciprocal coordination of one agonist muscle group and its antagonist, or opposing, muscle group, as is commonly produced when there is a faulty postural alignment. Factors such as muscle fatigue or muscle imbalance caused by poor conditioning habits are frequently to blame for strains. Muscle cramping that results from profuse sweating and mineral loss can produce muscle tears.

Muscle strain intensity, as with all acute injuries, can be graded according to standards of mild, moderate, and severe, or first, second, and third degree. In dancers the most common sites of strains are in the legs and lower trunk regions. However, strains can also occur in the shoulder girdle and the neck. *First-degree strains* are usually associated with mild spasm and soreness that are usually not noticed until the day following the injury. In most cases of mild strain, the causative factor is muscle spasm, and not tearing or overstretching of the tissue. In *second-degree strain* the dancer usually senses the muscle tissue giving way or tearing, followed by spasm, pain, weakness, and loss of function in the area. There may be a sharp pain or burning sensation immediately following the occurrence of this strain. Feeling, or palpating, the affected part discloses point tenderness accompanied by muscle contraction and swelling. When the tissue has been ruptured, an indentation may be felt. The *severe* or *third-degree strain* displays immediate severe pain, burning sensation, loss of function, and point tenderness. Whenever a third-degree strain is detected, especially if there is severe loss of function that lasts for a long time in the affected part, medical attention must be obtained immediately.

Sprain. Although probably less common in dance than the strain, a sprain is one of the most disabling injuries that can occur to the dancer. A sprain is a wrenching of a joint that produces a stretching or tearing of the joint's stabilizing connective tissue. When the joint is forced beyond its anatomical limits, the articular capsule, synovial membrane, and tendons can be adversely affected. The sprain is associated with varying degrees of joint swelling, tenderness, and loss of function and, like the contusion and strain, can be categorized as first, second, or third degree. The first-degree sprain involves slight stretching of the connective tissue with very little loss of function and perhaps a twinge of pain when the joint is twisted. The moderate sprain is much more severe, often taking up to 2 or 3 weeks to heal. The third-degree sprain is a serious condition and normally involves a great deal of swelling and loss of joint function. A third-degree sprain may be almost a dislocation of the joint.

Dislocation. A dislocation is a disunion of one bone in its relationship to another bone, resulting in extensive pathological damage. Dislocations may be divided into two types: partial dislocation, or *subluxation,* and complete dislocation, known as *luxation.* A dislocation must always be considered at least as serious as a fractured bone. Often associated with a joint disunion is a fracture that occurs because of the ripping away of supportive tissue. The dislocated joint is best recognized by its deformity; the dancer should be automatically referred to a physician for medical treatment.

Fracture. A fracture is a disruption of a bone's continuity. Although it is not as common as other internal conditions discussed, there are situations in which fractures can be incurred by the dancer. For example, the dancer can fall from a height, suddenly twist a part, or spontaneously fracture an area that has become overstressed or fatigued. In the most severe cases of fracture, jagged bone ends can protrude through the skin, causing both internal and external pathological damage. The dancer should note that all severe musculo-skeletal dance injuries should be considered fractures and routinely referred to a physician. Fracture signs are deformity, rapid swelling, extreme tender-ness at the site, and partial or complete loss of function. In some cases, a fracture site may appear as an extra joint and produce a grating sound when moved. All suspected fractures should be splinted, including the joints above and below the injury site, to ensure proper stabilization.

CHRONIC INJURIES

As discussed earlier, the acute injury is one that comes on suddenly and, if cared for properly, is resolved quickly. On the other hand, an acute injury that is not properly managed in its early stages or that is aggravated by repeated injury may become chronic. A chronic problem is defined as one that has a *gradual onset and long duration.* The chronic problem, whether it originates from a contusion, strain, or sprain, represents a constant irritation with a low-grade inflammatory state usually associated with a great deal of scarring. At all costs the dancer should avoid repeated injuries to any area in an attempt to prevent a chronic condition. The chronic problem is often named for the tissue that it is associated with, such as *bursitis, myositis, fasciitis, periostitis,* or *tendinitis.*

Once a chronic problem has been incurred, it must be cared for by conservative means. This usually includes rest and elimination of further aggravation combined with appropriate physical therapy and supportive procedures. The dancer should be apprised that once a chronic problem has been incurred, there is usually a tendency for recurrence under similar conditions.

INJURY INSPECTION AND EVALUATION

When injured, dancers frequently tend to ignore what the body is telling them about their injury. The myth that seems to permeate the dance profession is that pain must be expected and must be overcome by "dancing through the pain." As a result, acute injuries become chronic, and relatively mild problems become more serious. The extent of pain and loss of function are a dancer's best indication of the degree of injury. The reason for a hurt must be assessed. For example, superficial muscle pain stemming from hard work or perhaps overuse is a much different pain than that which may be sharp and deep, coupled with weakness in a given part. In the latter situation, immediate first-aid procedures of cold, compression, elevation, and rest are essential, as soon as possible. In the case of a chronic problem, there is a constant feeling of discomfort that may become lessened during activity and increased in severity at rest. Other indicators of injury are the more obvious symptoms of discoloration in the skin, swelling, and deformity. Also, the dancer might hear abnormal sounds on movement such as grating, sloshing, snapping, or cracking along with pain symptoms. Point tenderness also reflects a pathological condition in a particular area. Through feeling a site, a dancer is able to discern swellings, lumps, or other tissue disruptions not obvious to the eye. The fingertips can also determine whether the injury involves soft tissue or bony tissue.

SHOCK

When the musculoskeletal system is involved, shock must always be interpreted as a sign of severe injury. It is related to the injury proper and also to the psychological manifestations that often accompany a traumatic situation. Shock occurs as the result of a diminished amount of fluid in the circulatory system that inhibits red blood cells from adequately distributing oxygen throughout the body. When shock occurs, plasma (the fluid part of the circulatory system) disperses to the outside tissue spaces, leaving the solid particles within the blood vessels unable to flow adequately throughout the body. When shock occurs, blood pressure usually drops and the pulse becomes weak, shallow, and rapid, often causing the dancer to become lightheaded and nauseous. Any moderate to severe injury can bring about physiological shock; however, fear and emotional upset about an injury can also cause shock to happen.

Those helping the injured dancer should always expect shock when a serious injury is present and act accordingly. Under these circumstances the dancer should be maintained in a reclining position with the head and trunk level, the lower limbs elevated slightly, and the body temperature kept as normal as possible. For the highly sensitive individual who has a fear of injury or an extremely low pain threshold, it is desirable to keep spectators away and to keep an unsightly injury covered. Medical attention should be obtained as soon as possible.

10

Caring for the dance injury

Those who are involved with dance should have a basic understanding of how to manage first- and second-degree injuries. The dancer is capable of learning to provide self-care for less serious problems. The management of third-degree injuries, at least in their initial stages, must be undertaken by a physician. No injury need be neglected because of a lack of funds to receive care.

The purpose of this chapter is to give basic information on proper immediate and follow-up care, to present therapeutic approaches that are well within the capabilities of the dancer to administer, and to make the dancer more knowledgeable about what to expect from health professionals.

IMMEDIATE CARE

As stated earlier, in the initial stages of an acute musculoskeletal injury five major procedures are commonly performed: application of some cold medium, commonly ice; compression, usually by an elastic wrap; elevation; immobilization by a splint or some strapping technique, and appropriate rest. All of these procedures assist the body in confining hemorrhage, in reducing muscle spasm, and in generally organizing the injury of healing. The reader must remember that these procedures do not speed the healing process but make the best conditions for healing to take place. As long as the injury is still hemorrhaging and has not begun to organize, it must continue to be treated by appropriate immediate procedures ranging from as short as a half an hour to as long as 72 hours.

FOLLOW-UP CARE

Follow-up care implies all the procedures that are applied that assist in the healing process. Although the dancer typically is not a therapist, he or she can safely employ a great many therapy possibilities without extensive training. The purpose of this section is to present numerous superficial therapeutic techniques that can be chosen by the dancer and to provide an understanding of the deeper therapies that are commonly used by licensed health professionals. Therapeutic exercise is also discussed, as are practical supportive methods.

Cold (Cryotherapy)

Cold can be used as a follow-up therapy technique. It is becoming very popular as a therapeutic agent and is very often used in preference to heat.

The dancer will find cold application important in constricting superficial blood vessels and inhibiting local blood circulation immediately following an injury. Cold combined with compression and elevation of the part tends to localize internal hemorrhaging and helps in resolution of the injury. In terms of follow-up therapeutic care, ice is extremely valuable when a spasm is present. Cold application reduces spasm and the associate pain by reducing pressure on the pain receptors.[3]

Cold can be applied in many forms by the dancer (Fig. 10-1). Cold packs can be made by placing ice in a towel or, for the dancer who will be in a place where a cold medium is not available, a chemical cold pack can be purchased. Cold-water immersion with water temperatures of approximately 60°F is a good means of producing analgesia or inhibiting pain in the area.

A technique that has become popular in the care of muscle injuries is *ice massage* (Fig. 10-2). To perform ice massage, water is frozen in a paper cup and then the paper is torn off, producing a cylinder of ice. One thickness of a towel is wrapped around the ice, which is used to make small circular movements over the affected part until three important phases are experienced. Phase one is the sensation of cold; phase two is the sensation of mild aching, in which the skin turns a bright red; and phase three is the numbing stage. When the part has reached the numb stage it is put into a gradual stretch, which is maintained for 30 seconds to 1 minute. This cold stretch process is repeated several times a day. The ice massage technique helps to reduce muscle spasm as well as assisting the dancer in the mobilizing the injured part. Because it is readily accessible and inexpensive, ice massage is one of the most valuable cold therapy techniques.

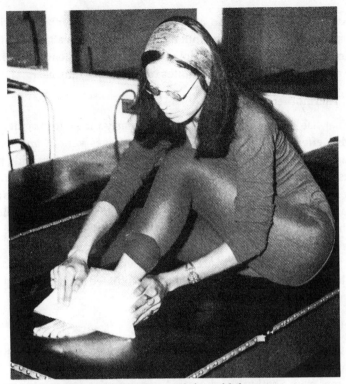

Fig. 10-1. Use of an ice pack for cold therapy.

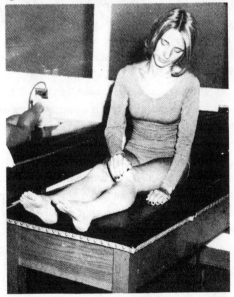

Fig. 10-2. Application of ice massage to a swollen knee.

An excellent addition to cold application is to combine it with mild exercise. Using cold exposure until numbness has been attained for at least 20 minutes, the dancer should move the injured part gently in a pain-free range of movement for 2 to 3 minutes or until pain returns.

Heat (Thermotherapy)

Heat has been used for therapy since early times. It provides a pain-reducing effect, speeds up circulation, encourages venous and lymphatic drainage, and speeds up metabolism, thus assisting in the healing process. Because of the soothing effect of heat when first applied, the dancer may prefer heat over cold therapy. It should be avoided where swelling is present or is produced. The two major areas of thermotherapy are superficial and deep heat therapy. Superficial heating occurs on the surface of the skin, in contrast to deep heating, which penetrates deep within the body's tissues. Deep heating is in the province of a licensed health professional. On the other hand, superficial heating can be safely initiated by the dancer if reasonable precaution is taken.

Superficial heat therapy

Superficial heat therapy comes in many forms. Probably the most common forms are the heat that is generated from an electric pad and the heat that comes from a bathtub or shower. A very popular device is the moist heat pad shown in Fig. 10-3. Unlike cold therapy, heat should never be applied to an injured part when hemorrhaging is still occurring. As mentioned earlier, sometimes as long as 3 days should elapse following an injury before heat is applied to an area. Heat therapy should start at lower temperatures and be gradually increased daily.

Immersion Baths. Immersion baths (soaks), in which the injured part is placed in warm water, can eventually reach temperatures as high as 120°F with immersion lasting for 10 to 30 minutes, depending on the individual's skin sensitivity. However, it is suggested that a soak bath start with temperatures around 90°F. An important type of immersion bath is the whirlpool, or hydromassage (Fig. 10-4). The whirlpool is one of the most popular forms of hydrotherapy. The whirlpool combines the heat and soothing effect of the water with an agitation or massage action that mildly increases circulation. Like the soak, the whirlpool should start out at lower temperatures; a good beginning is an initial exposure of no longer than 10 minutes at a temperature of 90°F. The whirlpool temperature should never be above 100° to 105°F and should last no longer than 10 to 20 minutes. If the body is fully submerged to the neck in the whirlpool tub, exposure should not exceed 10 minutes at 100°F.

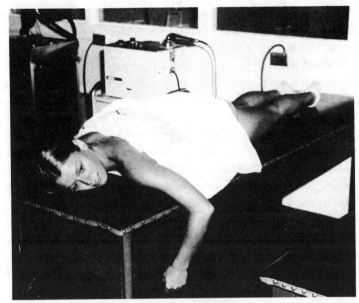

Fig. 10-3. Moist heat therapy.

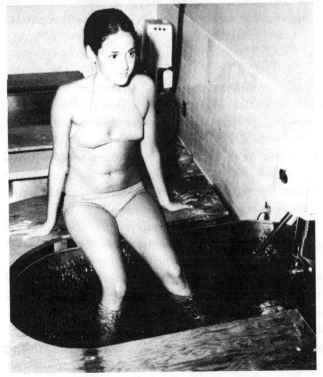

Fig. 10-4. Hydromassage in a whirlpool bath.

In the case of hydromassage, the jet stream should never be directed to the injured part but should be aimed at the side of the tub, with the circulation occurring secondarily around the injured member.

Contrast Baths. The contrasting technique, which alternates cold and hot water soaks, has been used for many years to relieve swelling and muscle spasm. This technique is excellent for injuries that are 3 or 4 days old and centered around major joints such as the ankle and knee. The dancer prepares two tubs of water, one with a temperature of 60°F and the other with a temperature of 105°F. The procedure starts with alternately soaking the part in the cold water for 2 minutes and in the hot tub for 5 minutes and then continuing to alternately soak the part 2 minutes in the cold water and 4 minutes in the hot. The entire contrast therapy regimen continues for approximately 30 minutes, with the last cycle finishing in the cold tub.

Many other superficial therapeutic heat techniques have proved to be beneficial. However, those that have been discussed are the most readily used by highly active people. Ideally, superficial heat as well as other therapy forms should be initiated two or three times daily. However, precautions must be taken against overexposing the injury to temperature extremes for long periods. For example, sensitive body tissue should always be protected by a cloth material before a hot pad or cold therapy is applied to the skin.

Deep heat therapy

It is readily apparent that a book of this type is not intended to give the reader definitive information on all physical therapy techniques. This is particularly true in the case of the deep heat therapies. It is important, though, that a dancer have some understanding of the deep therapies to appreciate the medical implications of their use.

The three most common deep heat modalities are shortwave, microtherm, and ultrasound diathermy. Shortwave and microtherm diathermy both use high-frequency electric current as a therapeutic aid (Fig. 10-5). Shortwave diathermy creates a nondirect and diffused heating of soft tissue, whereas microtherm diathermy creates a more direct heating of an area. On the other hand, ultrasound therapy consists of sound energy that is converted to heat energy (Fig. 10-6). Ultrasound must be applied to the injured area through a liquid medium such as mineral oil or water. In contrast to diathermy, ultrasound works most effectively on dense conective tissue, such as fascia and/ or ligaments. Muscle stimulation is widely used in the rehabilitation of injured muscles. Depending on the electric current used in physical therapy, varying physiological responses can be produced. An alternating (faradic) current produces an intermittent flow of electric current to the muscles and

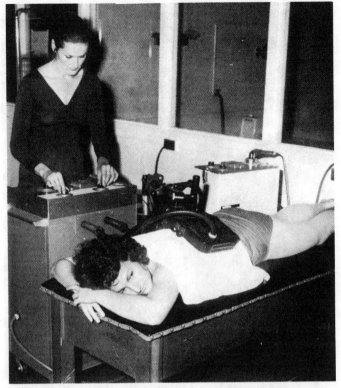

Fig. 10-5. Shortwave diathermy.

assists in preventing atrophy. The other commonly used current is sinusoidal, a gradual and rhythmical current with rising and falling intensity. It can produce mild exercise of a part as well as assist in relaxation of tense and fatigued muscles. However, muscle stimulation applied to the healthy individual with normal muscles that have become injured cannot be compared with active exercise for rehabilitation.

Analgesic balms and liniments

Although not actually a heat media, analgesic balms and liniments are often used to bring about much the same effect as superficial heat therapy. Both analgesic balms and liniments contain a rubefacient, a substance that provides a mild irritation to the skin. The rubefacients commonly found in analgesic balms are oil of wintergreen, red pepper, and menthol. The mild skin irritation that is created causes superficial capillaries to dilate, increasing circulation as well as countering the sense of mild pain such as may be

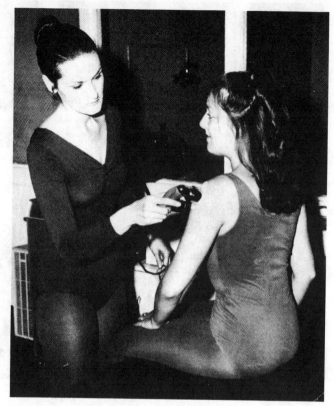

Fig. 10-6. Ultrasound therapy.

associated with muscle soreness. At no time should balms or liniments be used that contain anesthetic such as chloriform or procaine hydrochloride (Novacain). Unlike a skin analgesic, an anesthetic completely blocks pain and the dancer could sustain an even more serious injury.

Massage

Massage is one of the world's oldest therapeutic modalities. Most cultures, both ancient and modern, have employed this means as a health aid. The therapeutic massage most commonly used today in the United States has its origins in the work of Mitzger of Holland and Ling of Sweden. This massage is performed passively on the individual by another person; however, a person can also employ self-massage in some areas of the body. Massage is an inexpensive and readily available therapy technique. Physiologically, massage can encourage venous and lymphatic drainage, stretch soft tissue, increase nutrition and metabolism to a given area, and assist in removing waste products more readily. Depending on the technique employed, massage can relax or stimulate the body.

Many factors must be taken into consideration for effective massage. Most techniques of massage use a friction-proofing medium such as cold cream, mineral oil, or talc to prevent skin and hair from pulling. For effective massage, the body must be placed in a completely relaxed position. If the body is tense, the effect of the massage may be completely nullified.

The three most prevalent techniques used in massage therapy are effleurage, petrissage, and friction techniques.

Effleurage. Effleurage is either light or deep stroking (Fig. 10-7). Light stroking is designed to relax or bring about a sedative response. Deep stroking is designed to compress and to increase the venous and lymphatic circulation of the massaged part. Both types of effleurage may be used alternately on the dancer. Effleurage is applied differently to different parts of the body. For example, when stroking the back, the operator starts in the lower back region and moves upward along the spine to the top of the

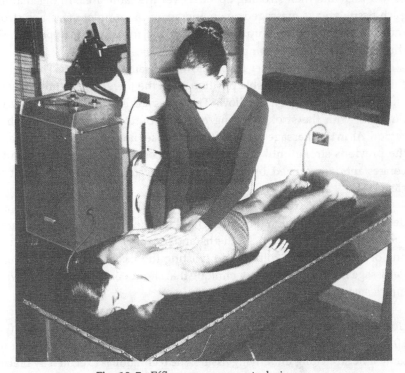

Fig. 10-7. Effleurage massage technique.

shoulders, applying constant pressure with the heels of the hands. When the hands have reached the top of the shoulders, they move outward from the spine about ½ inch on each side and then trail down, with the fingertips returning to the starting point. This procedure is continued until the hands have traveled the full width and length of the back. Then the hands are moved from the outside of the back inward, tracing the area of the back that has already been covered. In massaging the back the operator may also want to add a lift and roll when the trapezius muscle has been reached. This is known as trapezial milking. The effleurage stroke should be slow and rhythmical in every respect and should last no longer than 5 to 7 minutes on any given part of the body.

In the effleurage technique for the shoulder and arm, the dancer lies with the affected side facing the operator. In this position the affected shoulder or arm is relaxed and readily available for massage. The massage starts high up on the shoulder area, with the arm resting over the operator's shoulder. The operator's hands travel up over the top of the deltoid muscle, over the back of the scapula, and in front of the pectoralis area. The hands stroke upward and then trail downward, overlapping the proceeding stroke about ½ to 1 inch and then stroking upward over the same area. In this manner, each tissue area is massaged again and again. A complete massage stroke moves from the fingertips up and over the wrist, forearm, and upper arm and then over the shoulder complex.

Effleurage to the lower limb follows the same principles. The leg and thigh are put in a comfortable position, with the lower leg slightly elevated and the feet resting on a pillow. The massage is started just below the buttocks, with the stroke moving over the buttocks and the lower back region. As in the massage of the arm, each subsequent stroke is started below the previous stroke until the entire leg has been rubbed. In this manner, congestants are carried by the circulatory system back to the heart for cleansing.

Petrissage. Petrissage is therapeutic kneading designed to loosen and decongest a tissue region (Fig. 10-8). It is best executed in bulky tissue areas such as the trapezius, buttocks, thighs, and triceps. The massage technique is one of lifting, pulling, rolling, and twisting the tissue without pinching it. Petrissage is a fairly vigorous technique that should only be employed when injuries have been fully resolved.

Friction. Friction is an excellent technique for massaging body tissue closest to bone, such as around joints, and for relieving muscle spasms (Fig. 10-9). This technique is designed to increase local circulation while at the same time stretching underlying tissue. The technique is executed by bracing

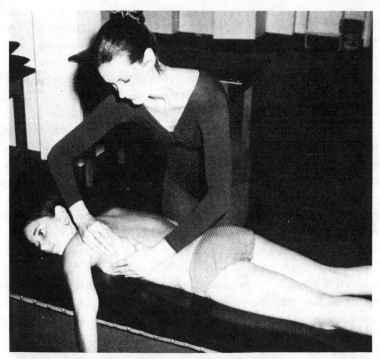

Fig. 10-8. Petrissage massage technique.

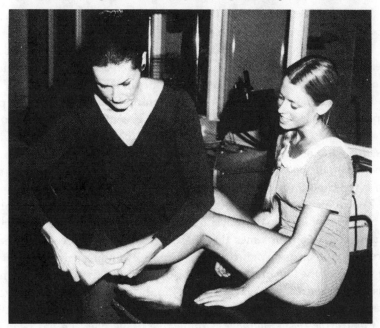

Fig. 10-9. Friction massage technique.

the heels of the hand while the fingers make circles in opposite directions. The fingers can also be braced to free the thumbs for massaging.

Effleurage, petrissage, and friction techniques are particularly applicable to the problems that face dancers. They can be employed easily by other dancers or in some cases by the dancer. (Purposefully not discussed here are the techniques of percussion or tapotement. Perscussion massage, which commonly includes the techniques of slapping, hacking, and cupping, is not considered therapeutic.) The dancer should be warned that massage is contraindicated when an injury is still hemorrhaging. If there is doubt about the resolution of an injury, massage should be applied above and below the injury site. When it is certain that the injury is not hemorrhaging, massage should begin over the injured site, lightly at first and then progressively harder.

Massage should never be used as a means to warm up in place of the regular active warm-up procedures. However, it is valuable as a means of stretching and loosening an injured area in conjunction with the warm-up regimen. A general body massage will assist the dancer who feels fatigue or stiffness due to congested muscles.

Other massage techniques used by dancers

Two less traditional forms of massage are reflex site determination and massage and deep connective tissue massage.

Reflex site determination and massage. The two areas of reflex site determination and massage that are becoming increasingly popular among dancers are shiatsu, or acupressure, and zone therapy, or reflexology.

In Japanese, shiatsu means finger pressure and it employs the concept of acupuncture and massage. It uses deep massage with the ball of the thumb and sometimes the thumbnail. Shiatsu subscribes to the idea that when pressure is applied to selected points on the body, symptomatic relief occurs elsewhere in the body. The pressure is firmly initiated for 5 to 7 seconds and then is repeated three to four times.[24]

Zone therapy, or reflexology, is a speciality of reflex point determination and massage confined to the foot and hand. Like ear acupuncture or auriculo-therapy, reflexology assumes that the outer surfaces of the foot or hand represent other areas on or in the human body. By finding pain points on the skin surface of the foot or hand, one may detect organ dysfunction. Then by massaging that area, one may give relief to the dysfunction. To date, zone therapy does not seem to be as well established as other reflex therapies.[17]

Connective tissue massage. Connective tissue massage has been becoming increasingly popular in the last few years, with two types being the most popular; namely, Elizabeth Dicke's *Meine Bindeqewebsmassage* (connective tissue massage) and Ida P. Rolf's structural integration (rolfing).

In Dicke's approach, connective tissue of the body is considered to be closely associated with metabolism, regulation of acid-base equilibrium, water content, salt content, and osmotic pressure regulation. The massage technique is performed by the operator's ring finger and middle finger of either hand, depending on what side of the body is being massaged. The fingers apply pressure to the skin so that it is stretched along with the subcutaneous tissue and the deeper fascia, composed of connective tissue. The stroking is done in different directions depending on the part of the body being massaged. A reflex action results from the pressure and deep pull of the tissue.

Structural integration, or rolfing, is a technique designed for realigning the major body segments. The primary tissue affected by faulty postural habit patterns is fascia. As a result of postural imbalances, it is believed that the body may reflect restricted movement, circulation impairment, and tonal imbalances in various musculature. Rolfing consists of a sequence of lengthening and centering activities that are designed to correct adverse postures. Rolfing takes place in a series of ten sessions lasting an hour each and spaced about a week apart. The practitioner applies a force hard enough to move underlying connective tissue. Often, pain is intense in the process but disappears immediately after the pressure is released. Residual soreness may last a few days. Rolfing is associated with emotional release as postural integration takes place.[11]

EXERCISE AND THE INJURY

Exercise properly executed is one of the most important therapeutic modalities. Two exercise considerations are important to the dancer who is attempting to recover from a musculoskeletal injury. These considerations are divided into a generalized exercise program and a specific therapeutic exercise program.

A general program of exercise should be instituted to prevent deconditioning that comes from inactivity. The reconditioning program following an injury includes exercising the entire body with the exception of the specific injured part, which is isolated from activity until it can engage in a specific therapeutic regimen. A dancer who suffers from a severe infection, is debilitated because of fatigue, or has some chronic inflammatory condition must avoid the general conditioning program. It is commonly known that prolonged inactivity results in a general lack of physical strength and in muscle atrophy. If confined to bed for a long time, the dancer will also experience a demineralization of bones. The reconditioning program should develop all the physical fitness attributes of strength, flexibility, endurance, and the maintenance of coordination without aggravating the injured part.

Following the initiation of a generalized exercise program, if the injured dancer is to return to full function as soon as possible, therapeutic exercise of the injured part should be initiated. However, the specific therapeutic exercises must not adversely affect the injury. Therapeutic exercises are applied as soon as the obvious acute stages, particularly pain, have diminished.

Therapeutic exercise, like the general exercise program, involves four primary factors: strength, flexibility, muscle endurance, and coordination. Each of these qualities must be restored to the part before the dancer may safely return to a full activity program. Reconditioning exercises will be discussed more fully in Part V.

SUPPORTIVE AND PROTECTIVE TECHNIQUES

It is important that a dancer have a working knowledge of the values and uses of various materials that can protect and support the body in an injury situation. The areas discussed in this book are thought to be the most important and practical to the dance field and include various types of bandages, adhesive tape, and padding techniques.

Bandages

The most common types of bandages used are the triangular, the cravat, and the roller bandage. The triangular and cravat bandages are used mainly in first-aid situations and most commonly in cases of arm or shoulder injuries. A cervical sling is made by positioning the triangular bandage under the injured arm with the apex facing the elbow (Fig. 10-10). The end of the triangle closest to the body is carried over the shoulder of the injured arm while the other end is allowed the hang down loosely. The loose end is then pulled over the shoulder on the uninjured side, and the two ends of the bandage are tied in a square knot behind the neck. The end of the bandage that sticks out at the elbow is then brought around to the side of the elbow and pinned.

The roller bandage, which can be made from different materials and in a variety of widths, is probably the most handy of the available types of bandages. It comes in gauze, cotton cloth, and elastic material as well as in many synthetic materials applicable to almost any part of the body.

Some general rules that apply to any type of roller bandage are as follows:

1. The roller bandage should be held in the preferred hand with the loose end extending from the bottom of the cylinder.

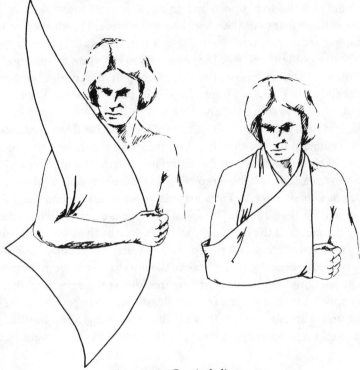

Fig. 10-10. Cervical sling.

2. Constant pressure should be applied on the bandage throughout the entire procedure.
3. The wrap must be tight enough to be held firmly in place but not so tight that it impedes circulation.
4. Each turn of the wrap should overlap at least half the width of the preceding turn, ensuring that the wrap will not separate and expose the skin.
5. Ideally, if the wrap is to cover a large area, it is best to start the wrap at the smallest circumference and wrap toward the largest circumference of the part.
6. The wrap should be secured by being tied or held firmly with adhesive tape; however, the end of the wrap should never be at the site of the injury.

Figure-of-eight, spica, and spiral bandages. Figure-of-eight and spica bandages are the most practical for active people. When elastic-wrap material is used, the figure-of-eight and spica serve to hold dressings in place, to provide mild soft-tissue support, and to allow for full movement by the individual without fear of the bandage becoming loose. The elastic bandage is sometimes used over a strapping technique to provide additional support. Both the figure-of-eight and spica are executed in the same manner, except that the spica has a larger loop on one end. Although spica or figure-of-eight bandages can be placed on any joint of the body, they are mainly used on the ankle, foot, hip, knee, shoulder, and elbow.

Ankle and foot spica (Fig. 10-11). A 2-inch elastic bandage is anchored around the metatarsal arch; then it is brought across the instep, around and behind the heel, and back across the instep to return to the metatarsal. This procedure is repeated with the wrap moved continuously upward until the entire foot has been covered. Extra material is wrapped around the ankle.

Spiral bandage (Fig. 10-12). The spiral bandage is used often in dance to assist with problems of the leg, thigh, and occasionally the lower and upper arms. The material of choice for the spiral is an elastic wrap between 2 and 3 inches in width, depending on the size of the area to be covered. The spiral bandage is anchored at the smallest circumference of the part and usually proceeds upward against gravity in a spiral fashion. When an elastic wrap is used, it is best to anchor the spiral by starting at one angle and then, as the wrap is brought around the part, changing the direction of the angle. In this

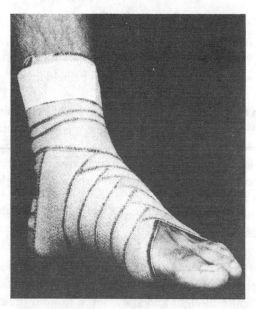

Fig. 10-11. Ankle and foot spica.

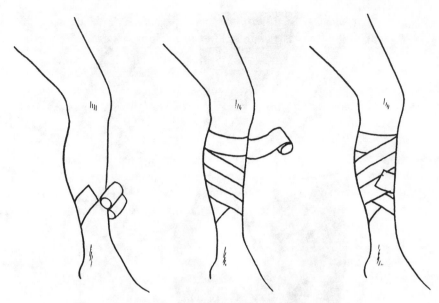

Fig. 10-12. Spiral elastic wrap technique.

manner the wrap will be firmly anchored and not slip as it continues upward above the injured site and then proceeds downward. A good rule of thumb in completing the spiral wrap is to never go down as far as the starting point and never go up as far as the end point but to concentrate the spirals in the center of the wrapped limb.

Knee figure-of-eight bandage. The knee is a difficult joint to wrap effectively. A spiral bandage is often preferred over the figure-of-eight because it is easier to apply and seems to stay in place better during activity. However, the figure-of-eight bandage is best used to secure a dressing on either the front or the back of the knee or when compression is near the kneecap or the back of the knee and around the thigh. It is subsequently carried downward, crossing the kneecap again. This procedure is continued until all the material has been applied.

Hip spica (Fig. 10-13). The hip spica is one of the most practical wraps used in dance. It serves to provide mild pressure and support to the hip and groin muscles as well as to efficiently hold a heat pad or ice pack over the injury site. Because of the limited amount of material, the hip spica technique must be well planned and executed. The end of a 6-inch elastic wrap is placed at a point on the upper thigh over the injured site. Anchoring is initiated at a point on the upper thigh over the injured site by encircling the thigh, moving up the thigh to the groin, across the lower abdominal area, and around the

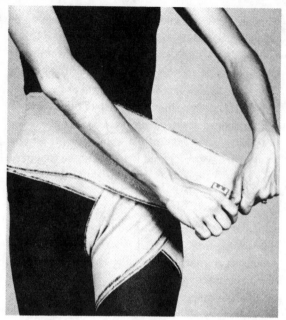

Fig. 10-13. Hip spica.

crest of the ilium. The wrap is then continued around the lower back and crossed over the thigh.

Shoulder spica (Fig. 10-14). Although used less commonly than the other figure-of-eight and spica wraps mentioned, the shoulder spica is a technique that dancers will need if a strain of the shoulder occurs and a mild support is needed. Before the shoulder is wrapped, the underarm should be well padded to prevent constriction of blood vessels. The wrap starts at the midpoint of the deltoid region and proceeds around in back of the underarm, in front of the deltoid, around the back underneath the unaffected arm, and around the chest to the starting point. In wrapping of the shoulder it is imperative that the dancer maintain good posture, holding the shoulders in proper alignment.

Elbow figure-of-eight bandage (Fig. 10-15). Like the shoulder spica, the elbow figure-of-eight will only occasionally be needed. It is similar in pattern to the knee figure-of-eight, the bandage being anchored by encircling the lower arm with one complete turn. It then crosses either in front of or in back of the elbow and proceeds upward to encircle the upper arm one complete turn. The pattern is continued with the wrap always moving toward the center of the joint, ending at the upper arm area.

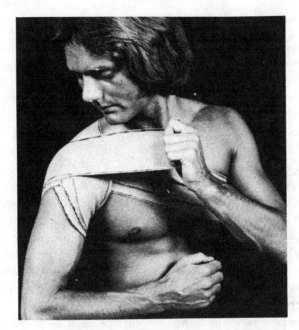

Fig. 10-14. Shoulder spica.

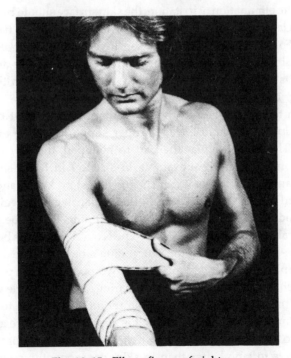

Fig. 10-15. Elbow figure-of-eight.

Adhesive tape

Adhesive tape is being used increasingly in the prevention and protection of injuries to active people. There are a great many types of adhesive tape now available. The two most popular types are rigid nonyielding linen-backed tape and elastic tape. Both have special importance in the prevention and care of injuries. In recent years the production of special lightweight athletic tape has become a boon to active people. Many of these tapes on the market are both lightweight and strong. Three features make up the best quality of athletic tape: backing, mass, and unwinding properties. When properly applied, the lightweight tape can provide a high degree of strength and protection for the dancer and is much preferred over heavier tape. For the person who is going to wear tape for a long time, it is important that the adhesive mass be of high quality, having the ability to resist profuse perspiration, body heat, and movement. The tape mass must not irritate the skin or leave a residue on the skin when removed. It is also important that tape unwind evenly throughout the entire roll. It is difficult, if not impossible, to properly apply tape that has variable unwinding qualities.

Before tape is applied, the skin surface must be properly prepared. Perspiration and dirt as well as hair must be removed. For good tape adherence and the elimination of irritation, the skin surface should be sprayed with a commercial tape adherent that provides a tacky residue and has toughening qualities. For skin that is extremely sensitive to tape or for skin areas that must remain taped for a long time, there is now available an underwrap material that provides a thin yet snugly fitting covering on the skin to be taped (Fig. 10-16).

When tape is applied to the body, many factors must be taken into consideration in order to ensure proper support and the elimination of irritation. The more angular the part to be taped, the narrower the tape should be and vice versa. For example, ½-inch to 1-inch tape should be used for hands and feet, whereas 1½-inch tape is best for knees, and 2-inch tape can be used for the lower back and other expansive both regions. In cases where a body part is to be supported by strapping, it must be placed in the most neutral position possible. When tape is overlapped, it is best to overlap at least one-half the width of the proceeding tape layer. The dancer should note that tape must never be continuously wrapped around a part but should be torn each time a circle is executed. Tearing after each circle avoids losing control of the tape and prevents application that might be too tight. Tape should be molded and smoothed as it is applied, once piece at a time. It is desirable to allow the tape to conform to the natural contours of the body. Tape adheres to tape better than to skin; consequently, most techniques

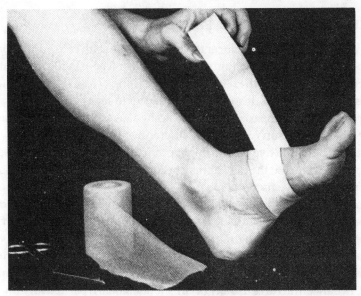

Fig. 10-16. Protective underwrap material for skin protection during strapping.

employed in taping should have an anchor strip at the beginning and a lock strip after application of a particular pattern. Although there are many types of underwraps (such as gauzes, pads, stockinettes, and prewrap materials), the dancer should realize that the best support is afforded by tape applied directly over skin.

Padding

There are many protective and supportive devices available to the dancer other than bandages and adhesive tapes. These devices can be purchased commercially, or they can be constructed out of a variety of materials. In dance, padding is primarily used for foot problems and is designed to brace, protect, or reestablish normal weight bearing. The most common materials used are moleskin (felt with an adhesive mass backing), sponge (with an adhesive backing), and podiatrist felt (⅛-inch felt material that also has an adhesive backing). In most cases pads should be custom-made, because commercial pads are not usually sufficiently durable to withstand the great forces that are produced by the dancer. Caution should be taken that the wearing of commercial orthopedic pads or braces does not force the dancer's body out of normal postural balance. If this does occur, other tissue breakdown may be expected in other parts of the body. More details will be given on specific protective and supportive devices in Part V.

DANCERS AND HEALTH CARE PROFESSIONALS

It is often difficult for the dancer to know when a health care professional should be contacted following injury. Fear of pain or fear of being kept out of dance activity often causes the dancer to wait too long before seeking professional help. Therefore, it is desirable for the dancer to seek help from a health professional who empathizes with the physically active individual. Obviously the active, healthy person reacts much differently to an injury than one who is sedentary. The less-active person might profit by many days or even weeks of conservative care, but the dancer may become psychologically depressed by long periods of inactivity.

In cases of musculoskeletal injury, an X-ray may be warranted to discount the possibility of fracture. X-ray examinations are routine for injuries of the joints because of the high probability of fracture in those areas. Even though an X-ray film cannot indicate or detect ligamentous tears, it can show the amount of abnormal laxity present in a particular joint when the joint is stressed. In dance, fractures usually occur spontaneously, particularly under fatigue conditions. Muscles can also pull alway pieces of bone if a contraction is strong enough. In both instances, X-ray examination could determine the extent of injury.

Therapeutic systems

In general there are two major therapeutic systems under which a doctor may practice. These are allopathy and naturopathy. Allopathy is a healing system that treats disease by producing a second condition that is antagonistic to the disease being treated. Naturopathy, on the other hand, is a therapeutic system that does not use drugs but confines practice to natural means such as light, heat, air, water, massage and/or manipulation as well as proper nutrition. Examples of allopathic professions are medical, osteopathic, and podiactric physicians. In contrast, chiropractors are naturopaths.

Medicine. Medicine refers to treatment of a disease medically with a drug or other agents as opposed to employing surgery. Medical doctors and osteopaths fall in this category. These doctors are generally known as physicians.

In the field of medicine there are numerous specializations. The first person a dancer sees is usually a family physican or person specializing in primary care. This person's responsibility is for initial screening, care of common illnesses, and health maintenance. If the dancer has a more or less serious musculoskeletal condition referral to an orthopedic surgeon may be appropriate.

The orthopedic surgeon deals with conditions of the musculoskeletal system. Disorders of the bones, joints, muscles, fascia, ligaments, and cartilage are remediated.

Osteopathy. Osteopathy, in contrast to chiropractic, belongs to the drug-using professions. Since the inception of osteopathy in 1870, skeletal manipulation has been a major part of its treatment regimen. According to osteopathy, carefully prescribed and applied manipulation helps correct acute and chronic postural and neuromusculoskeletal stress by the reduction of muscular tension, improving joint motion, relieving pressure or congestion around nerve roots, and determinig and blocking myofascial trigger point areas.[7] Modern osteopaths, whose education is comparable to that of the medical doctor, use drugs, surgery, and physical therapy, but still employ manipulation as an adjunct to their practice of medicine.

Chiropractic. Chiropractic falls under the category of natural healing in which no drugs are used. It employs procedures of diet and food supplementation along with spinal manipulation and physical therapy. Chiropractors operate on the theory that spinal subluxations, or misalignments, can cause unlimited problems to the neuromusculoskeletal system, adversely affecting organs and organ systems of the body. Manipulation of the spine, known as adjustment, is designed to realign subluxated vertebrae and thus normalize body functions, a belief that is vigorously challenged by medical doctors.

Podiatrics. Increasingly podiatrists are treating dancers. The field of podiatry is a health profession concerned with examination, diagnosis, injury prevention, and treatment of the human foot. Depending upon the state in which podiatry is practiced, the podiatrist can perform surgical procedures, prescribe corrective foot devices, and prescribe drugs as well as carry out physical therapy when required.

Conventional therapists

The two therapy fields most closely associated with dancers are physical therapy and athletic training.

Physical therapy. Physical therapy is therapeutic approach that is concerned with restoring musculoskeletal function through exercise, heat, cold, electricity, ultraviolet light, and massage and, in some cases, manipulation. Under the guidance of a physician the physical therapist carries out a treatment regimen, establishes provisions for further complications and, when applicable, trains the patient in activities of daily living.

Athletic training. On some occasions an athletic trainer may treat the dancer. This is particularly true in the college or university setting, or in a sports medicine clinic. The certified athletic trainer is skilled in aspects associated with the physically active individual such as the athlete and/or dancer, some of which are injury prevention, injury recognition and evaluation, injury treatment and referral, as well as in exercise rehabilitation.

Unconventional therapies and movement approaches

Dancers often gravitate to unconventional therapies and movement approaches in the hopes of maximizing efficient patterns of movement along with integrating the mind and body.

Acupuncture. Developed in China thousands of years ago acupuncture has become a major healing system. Needles are applied in specific skin sites that relate to certain body functions and organs. When the technique first appeared, stone needles the size of a small pencil were used to penetrate the body. Today, needles are made of very thin stainless steel.

The theoretical basis behind acupuncture is likened to a dual flow of energy known as yin and yang. Yin and yang are conceived together as the energy known as Ch'i or life force.[18] Yin and yang are opposite to one another and together produce a balance; yang tends to stimulate while yin sedates and calms. Within the body these opposite energies circulate along twenty-six meridians, each of which relates to a different body function. In recent years electro and laser stimulation has been added to the acupuncturist's repetoire.

Yoga as therapy. Yoga began in India over 6,000 years ago. Its main goal is to maintain healthy minds in healthy bodies. Although it is used to remediate illnesses, yoga goes beyond being a health system. Practitioners of yoga believe that most illness is produced by incorrect posture, wrong diet, and improper mental attitudes. Through the practice of meditation and hathayoga, in which specific postures are engaged in, physical and mental health is attained.[11]

T'ai Chi Ch'uan. T'ai Chi Ch'uan dates from about the first century A.D.. It was developed as an exercise system by a Taoist hermit who after long hours of sitting while meditating performed a series of movements to increase his circulation.[5] Movements were inspired by nature and are based upon the motions of birds, animals, streams, clouds, and the wind. T'ai Chi Ch'uan employs a routine of continuous relaxed flowing movement that encourages the balancing of Chi energy.

Body works/therapies

In the later part of this century a number of movement systems have come on the scene that are intended to alter the body's motor programming and thereby develop more fluency and efficiency in adapting to environmental forces, such as gravity, or internal stressors, such as anxiety. These systems help to repattern and integrate healthy habitual movement patterns that are applicable to activities of daily living as well as dance. Many of these systems are considered to have therapeutic attributes, but those who use these methods are not considered therapists but instructors. Some of the body works systems currently popular among dancers are Feldenkrais Method of Functional Integration, Alexander Method, Pilates Method, and the Juliu Horvath's Gyrotonic Expansion System.

Feldenkrais Method of Functional Integration. The Feldenkrais Method uses repetitive motion. At first the movement is slow and gentle, speeding up gradually, and finally slowing down again. The purpose is to increase self-awareness. As with all body works systems there is no body/mind dichotomy. By altering the body's motor patterns, the motor cortex is also altered. Through the engagement of habitual and nonhabitual movements, body awareness is increased and faulty movements patterns can be positively changed.[11]

Pilates Method. Developed in the early 1900s, Pilates Method employs exercises performed on a mat and on various types of apparatus (Fig. 10-17). The major piece of apparatus is the reformer, a horizontal platform with a movable carriage. Variable resistance is afforded the carriage by four detachable springs.

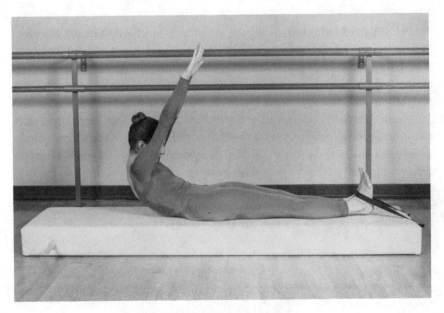

Fig. 10-17. Universal reformer.

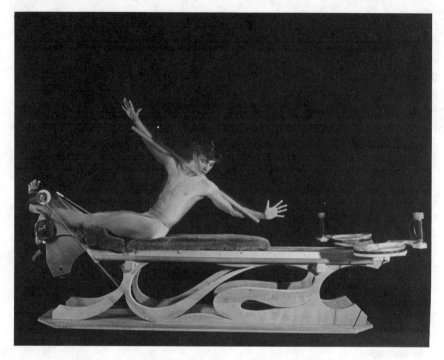

Fig. 10-18. Gyrotonics Expansion System.

The Pilates Method is used by the individuals, primarily dancers, desiring to enhance their dance training or who wish to supplement injury rehabilitation. Using the Pilates apparatus in rehabilitation assists the dancer in reestablishing or retaining patterns of movement without bearing weight. Each program is individually based.

Juliu Horvath's Gyrotonics Expansion System. The Gyrotonics Expansion System employs a series of sophisticated exercise machines developed with the dancer in mind. The system is designed to develop the dancers strength, flexibility, agility, balance, and centeredness. Using the principles of yoga, Gyrotonics emphasizes body perception and creativity. As with other body work systems, conditioning may prevent injuries or act to rehabilitate them when they occur (Fig. 10-18).

V

MUSCULOSKELETAL CONDITIONS COMMON TO DANCE

Their prevention, recognition, evaluation, and management

Part V is concerned with the most prevalent conditions that occur in dancers. The following chapters give up-to-date information on the prevention and care of injuries resulting from physical forces that overly compress or stretch tissue. Specifically, compression, friction, strain, sprain, dislocation, and fracture injuries are discussed.

11

Compression and friction problems

Traumatic compression of tissue or friction is a common occurrence for the active person. Either striking with the body itself or being hit by some outside source can cause tissue to be contused. Compression of the tissue can be a single event, causing acute inflammatory conditions with hemorrhage, pain, swelling, and malfunction, or the result of repeated traumatic events, causing a chronic irritation such as that produced by abnormal pressures of poorly fitting shoes or the chronic compressions that come from faulty body alignment. Friction injury usually results from the resistance produced when the skin is rubbed against clothing or within shoes or when the skin comes in direct contact with the floor.

CONTUSIONS

Contusions (Table 8) or bruises that arise from a blow to the body can occur to any part of the dancer's anatomy. However, they most often happen in the leg or foot region. The body's reaction to contusion is dependent on the body site and its particular sensitivity. Extremely sensitive body areas are located on the inner thigh, the face, the shin, the heel, and any bony protuberances. The most resilient soft tissue, such as is found in the thigh region and the calf, can withstand a greater blow than, for example, the shin or the heel of the foot.

Generally speaking, contusions can be classified as first, second, and third degree. The first-degree, or mild, contusion has symptoms of minimal

Table 8. Acute contusion management

Degree of injury	Basic signs	Management phase	Treatment program			
			Physical therapy	Dosage	Reconditioning	Dosage
First degree	*Mild* blow to the body from an outside source causing abnormal tissue compression with little pathological damage; some muscle spasm may be present	Step 1: immediate care	1. Cold, pressure if pain symptoms last more than a few minutes	$^1/_2$-1 hr	1. Gradual stretch following cold and pressure and ROM (range of movement) exercises	Symptomatic
Second degree	*Moderate* blow to the body resulting in a bruise with pain, loss of function, point tenderness, and muscle spasm lasting from several minutes to several hours;	Step 1: immediate care	1. Cold, pressure; 20 min on, 20 min off 2. Elevation 3. May warrant referral to physician for medication	24-48 hr 24 hr	1. Gradual stretch following application of cold and ROM exercises	2-3 min twice daily

swelling and discoloration may occur if proper immediate treatment is not given				
Step 2: second day	1. Start program of gradual heating with warm water soak (100° F) or whirlpool (90° F) 2. Wear elastic wrap for support	15 min twice daily	1. Avoid activity of part until hemorrhage has ceased 2. Continue gradual stretch and ROM exercises 3. General body exercise without aggravation of injury	Twice daily
Step 3: third or fourth day	1. Superficial and deep heat may be applied, e.g., water soak (110° F) or whirlpool (102° F) 2. Deep heat, e.g., diathermy or ultrasound 3. Wear elastic wrap 4. If spasm and pain are present use ice massage 5. Analgesic balm pack	20 min three times daily As prescribed Three times daily When active	1. Gradually begin to exercise injury while wearing elastic wrap for muscle stability; do not exercise if pain is present 2. Dancer is sufficiently recovered when part is pain free	Three times daily

Continued.

Table 8. Acute contusion management—cont'd.

Degree of injury	Basic signs	Treatment program				
		Management phase	Physical therapy	Dosage	Reconditioning	Dosage
Third degree	*Severe* blow to the body resulting in extreme pain, loss of function, point tenderness, and muscle spasm lasting for several hours or longer; swelling and discoloration are common even with proper immediate care	Step 1: immediate care	1. Cold, pressure; 20 min on, 20 min off 2. Elevation of part 3. Refer to physician for examination and medication 4. Wear elastic wrap for compression	48-72 hr 24 hr	1. Gradual stretch *only* after a 24-hr period has passed	2-3 min twice daily
		Step 2: third or fourth day	1. Start gradual heat program with warm water soak (100° F) or whirlpool (90° F), contrast bath 2. Continue to wear elastic wrap	15 min twice daily	1. Do not exercise injured part 2. General exercise 3. Gradual stretch and ROM exercises after therapy	Twice daily
		Step 3: fourth or fifth day	1. See step 3 of second-degree contusion		1. Dancer has recovered sufficiently when part is pain free and has regained full strength and flexibility	

pain and some point tenderness lasting for a very short time. Consequently, the first-degree contusion normally produces little inflammation, with most of the discomfort, if any, coming from muscle spasm. To avoid swelling and discoloration, the dancer should apply an ice pack and elastic wrap for the remainder of the day. It is doubtful that a first-degree contusion would prevent the dancer from continuing activity the next day. If some swelling and irritation are apparent the next day, it is advisable to continue cold and pressure.

The second-degree, or moderate, contusion is caused by a hard blow to the muscle tissue or bone, resulting in an immediate loss of function with a great deal of pain and tenderness upon palpation or touch. This degree of contusion, if occurring to very soft tissue, may cause an immediate swelling and perhaps discoloration the next day. Much of the discomfort comes from muscle spasm in the area. Immediate treatment should consist of cold and pressure by an elastic wrap applied intermittently for at least 24 to 48 hours. Elevation of the part may also be advisable if rapid swelling and discomfort are present. When muscle spasm is evident, the affected muscle should be placed in a static or gradual stretch position and the position maintained for at least 1 hour. If there is extreme loss of function, it may be advisable to refer the injury to a physician for possible nonsteroidal anti-infammatory medication. If hemorrhage appears to be under control by the following day, a gradual program of heat therapy may be initiated. It is advisable that water-soak, therapy with temperatures not to exceed 90°F, be applied until the injury has ceased hemorrhaging. Following cold therapy, a very mild gradual stretch program will help alleviate muscle spasm and pain in the area. In cases where the moderate contusion causes the dancer to miss class for a number of days, it is advisable that a general exercise program be instituted to prevent deconditioning. However, exercising the contused area should be avoided until it is symptom-free. If the dancer needs to move the injured part, an elastic wrap should be worn to prevent clot disruption and re-hemorrhaging in the area. Therapeutic heat temperature should be gradually raised daily until whirlpool baths have reached 105°F. If water soaks are the treatment chosen, the temperature can be gradually raised to 110°F.

A third-degree contusion results from a severe and penetrating blow to the body. The result of this violent blow is extensive compression of soft tissue, producing muscle spasm and severe loss of function with extensive hemorrhaging and swelling. Because of the seriousness of this injury, a physician should be contacted to discount the possibility of fracture or muscle rupture. As in the moderate contusion, medication may be the choice of the physician for combating spasm and encouraging the speedy absorption of fluids associated with the injury. Immediate care includes cold, pressure, and elevation for up to 3 days or until hemorrhaging has fully ceased. Care is then similar to care of the moderate contusion: gradual heating is instituted and a graduated program of exercise is also begun.

Heel bruise

Calcaneal periostitis, or heel bruise, is one of the most handicapping acute injuries occurring to the active person. It is normally caused by stepping on a small object, overly compressing the tissue covering the heel bone (calcaneus), or by an abnormal shearing action of the skin covering the calcaneus. Some individuals are susceptible to the heel bruise because they have an irregularly shaped calcaneus. Because the dancer is unable to withstand the stresses of severe compression, whatever the cause, the heel bruise presents extreme pain and discomfort and, in many cases, completely prevents the dancer from placing the heel on the floor. Ideally, if a heel bruise is sustained, a cold compress should be applied immediately. However, it is discouraging to note that the heel bruise does not respond readily to most physical therapy procedures. If not reaggravated, this injury is self-limiting and will normally resolve itself in time. Because the dancer is usually unable to avoid weight bearing, in the case of heel bruise a protective strapping or padding should be applied to the heel region in an attempt to take the painful pressure off the bruise.

Various techniques can assist the dancer who is prone to heel bruises or who is experiencing one, such as the application of a doughnut cut from sponge rubber to assist in the equalization of pressures around the bruise and the application of a supportive strapping. The heel bruise strapping technique uses either 1- or ½-inch linen tape that is patterned into a basketweave cap around the heel (Fig. 11-1). The first piece of tape is placed at the base of the Achilles tendon, extending past both the internal and external ankle bones. The next tape piece is applied to the bottom of the heel, encircling it on both sides and finishing at the ends of the first strip. Tape is applied alternately until a complete cap has been applied to the heel.

Metatarsal bruise

A second site where bone bruises are prevalent is at the center of the metatarsal arch. Dancers who place a great deal of pressure on the ball of the foot often cause a bruise in this area. This problem is accentuated by a fallen metatarsal arch because weight bearing, instead of being on two points of the ball joint, is abnormally applied to three sites. The fallen metatarsal arch is prone to bruising when there is abnormal pressure as occurs in stepping on a small hard object. Another site for bruising is the second metatarsal, because of the condition of Morton's toe. In general, the metatarsal bruise can be relieved by a pad placed at the base of the metatarsal arch (Fig. 11-2). The

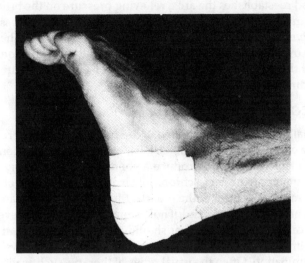

Fig. 11-1. Heel cap with 1-inch tape.

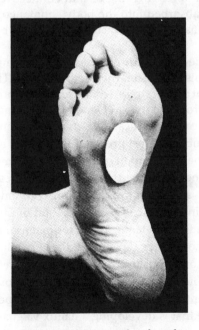

Fig. 11-2. Metatarsal arch pad.

metatarsal pad reestablishes the arch, relieving pressure on the bruise area. A pad can be made from many different materials but is most successful with either adhesive felt, ¼-inch thick, or adhesive sponge rubber. The dancer should cut an oval approximately 1½ inches in diameter and position the pad at the base of the metatarsal arch with a piece of 1-inch tape encircling the foot and holding the pad in place.

CHRONIC COMPRESSION PROBLEMS

Abnormal pressure can be applied to the body in many different ways that result in a chronic condition (Table 9). For example, repeated contusions at a particular muscle site can produce a condition known as *myositis ossificans*. In its attempt to protect a chronically irritated bruise, the body reacts by creating a mineral deposit in the muscle. Myositis ossificans can cause a great deal of pain for the dancer and, if not properly resolved, may eventually require surgical removal. The dancer should note that any bruise that does not respond immediately to therapy should be referred to a physician for complete examination. Often the usual types of therapy, such as ultrasound and massage, only serve to irritate and increase the mineral deposits when myositis ossificans is present. X-ray examination will reveal mineral deposits 2 or 3 weeks after the initial injury.

Occasionally when a bruise has occurred to the soft musculature, a hematoma, or bloom tumor, occurs within the muscle. A hematoma has a center of blood with an outer covering of thin connective tissue. A large hematoma often is not absorbed into the body spontaneously and consequently may have to be aspirated or evacuated medically by a hypodermic needle.

Compression injuries can occur chronically when improper postural alignment is present. This is particularly true in the feet. The dancer's feet normally undergo a great deal of stress, which can be compounded by faulty dance technique or improper footwear. Generally speaking, shoes that are too narrow or too short cause the toes to be cramped, eventually resulting in toe deformity. Toe problems most prevalent in dancers are bunions and the clawed or hammer toe. The bunion of the first or fifth metatarsal causes the great toe or the little toe to be forced toward the other toes. As a result, the joints become inflamed and often swollen from constant irritation. The clawed or hammer toe, in contrast, occurs as a result of the contraction of the toe flexor tendons and the stretching of the toe extensor tendons caused by shoes that are too short. Once developed, these conditions cannot be corrected by exercise or other positive means but can be relieved by strapping (Fig. 11-3). Bunions also produce inefficient movement and, if continually irritated, eventually require surgery. Tape properly applied can help stabilize a great toe that is developing a hallux valgus (Fig. 11-4).

Table 9. Chronic compression condition management

Common conditions	Basic signs	Treatment program					
		Management phase	Physical therapy	Dosage	Reconditioning	Dosage
Myositis ossificans	Ossification within a muscle caused by contusion that fails to respond to normal treatment and is marked by pain and swelling; x-ray examination may not show ossification until 2 or 3 weeks after injury	Symptomatic	1. Avoid massage 2. Apply superficial heat, e.g., whirlpool (102° F) 3. Mild gradual stretch of part 4. Protective strapping or pad 5. Anti-inflammatory medication	Two or three times daily Two or three times daily As prescribed	1. Avoid all exercise that may irritate part 2. Gradual stretch	Two or three times daily
Myositis, fasciitis, and periostitis	Continuous low-grade inflammation in tissue with mild swelling and pain; often most severe following activity	Symptomatic	1. Application of superficial and deep heat 2. Ice massage 3. Protective strapping or padding 4. Anti-inflammatory medication	Two or three times daily Twice daily As prescribed	1. Rest part when possible 2. Gradual stretch of part following ice massage	Twice daily

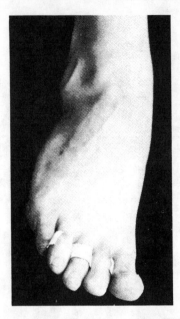

Fig. 11-3. Clawed or hammer toe strapping.

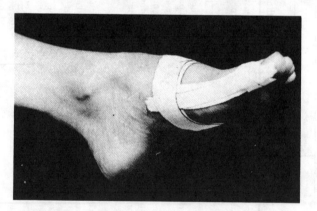

Fig. 11-4. Hallux valgus strapping.

The young dancer who goes on pointe before the feet are strong enough to maintain the foot, ankle, and leg in good alignment may develop deformities of the toes, particularly the great toe. The young child, therefore, should avoid going on pointe until the factors of weight, age, posture, and habits of body placement have been seriously considered.

Another problem of the great toe is the hallux rigidus. Although concerned with the great toe, the hallux rigidus is not a displacement, as is the bunion. The second joint of the great toe becomes extremely inflamed and painful in a straightened position, and gradually over a long period the toe becomes permanently rigid.

Constant abnormal pressure on the feet can lead to the development of painful calluses and extra bone growths, or bone spurs. Constant pressure breaks down tissue and is eventually reflected in a chronic disabling problem. Feet, in general, respond well to treatment of chronic inflammatory conditions by a regimen of repeated soaks two or three times daily in water that is 110°F. In situations where there is localized swelling and edema, contrast baths may be effective.

CHRONDROMALACIA

Chrondromalacia is the technical term for the softening of any cartilage. It occurs in dancers particularly in the knee joint and most frequently on the articular surface of the kneecap, which is composed of hyaline cartilage. Although the exact cause is unknown, abnormal compression forces, such as those created by abnormal postural alignment of the leg or repeated traumatic occurrences due to kneeling, seem to be precursors of the condition. Often associated with chrondromalacia is osteochondritis dissecans, a condition in which fragments of cartilage and underlying bone become detached from the articular surface and are free to move around in the joint space, causing noise in the joint and restriction of movement. The dancer who has these symptoms should be referred immediately to a physician for examination. Often this condition precludes physical activity for an extended period.

CALLUSES

Because they are on their feet a great deal, dancers often have calluses and/or blisters. These are caused by the skin of the feet shearing against the supportive surface. Contrary to common thinking, it is not desirable for a foot to have excess calluses. The cause of callus accumulation is often poor posture and weight bearing combined with faulty foot apparel. Callus accumulation reflects abnormal skin stresses and can result in an extremely painful condition of cracking and torn skin. A callus is tissue that is inelastic and has lost its viable yellow elastic tissue that is normally present in the subdermal skin layer. Having lost this elasticity, the callus moves as a mass and is vulnerable to tears and fissures.

Proper foot hygiene helps prevent callus formation. This is best accomplished by good dance technique, correct body alignment, the wearing of properly fitting footwear, and a good hygiene regimen that is followed several times a week. After dance class or rehearsal it is desirable for the feet to be cleansed thoroughly, followed by a routine of filing off of excess callus accumulation with an emery file and application of a very small amount of lanolin, which is massaged into the devitalized callus tissue (Fig. 11-5).

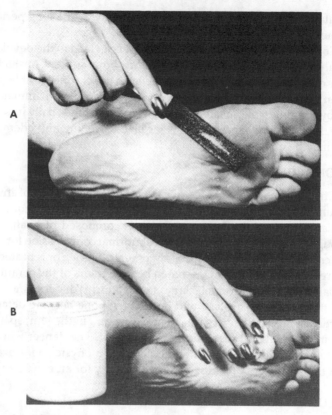

Fig. 11-5. A, Filing calluses. **B,** Applying lanolin to devitalized skin areas.

The dancer who senses abnormal friction on the foot should stop activity promptly and immediately give care to that area. Preventive care consists of eliminating irritation by friction-proofing the area. This can be done by rubbing it with petroleum jelly or padding it with a moleskin or tape covering that has been blanked out by placing a nonadhering piece of linen tape next to the side that will lie next to the irritation. A strategically placed adhesive-backed pad can also help take pressure off a painful callus (Fig. 11-6).

FRICTION BLISTERS

Like calluses, friction blisters result either from an excess of rubbing within a shoe or from skin rubbing against a nonyielding surface such as a stage or studio floor. Whatever the cause, the result of sustained friction is a separation of epidermis from the dermal skin layer with serum fluid accumulation under the epidermis. The fluid can be a clear serous material or can contain blood, depending on the depth of the tissues involved. The dancer

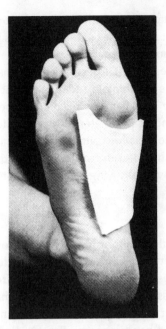

Fig. 11-6. Pad to relieve friction on the ball of the foot.

does well to prevent blisters from occurring. This, like callus prevention, must be started when the skin is first irritated. At that time either a friction-proofing substance such as petroleum jelly or protection from a medium such as moleskin or a blanked-out piece of tape should cover the irritated area.

Once a blister has developed, the dancer must prevent infection while at the same time engaging in full activity. Whenever possible, the dancer with a blister should follow a conservative approach in its management to ensure that infection does not arise. If the blister is located in such a place on the foot that it could be easily irritated by additional friction, it is desirable to evacuate the fluid with a sterilized needle. Sterilization can be accomplished by burning the needle tip with match and then cleansing the skin surface of the blister with rubbing alcohol. Following sterilization, the needle is introduced gently underneath the skin of the blister from about ⅛ inch outside the perimeter of the blister, tunneling under the blister until the fluid flows out. After evacuation, the blister should be protected by a felt or sponge rubber doughnut placed around the outside of the blister. Protected in this manner, the blister is allowed to heal. When it is no longer sensitive, the skin may be cut away from the area and allowed to toughen naturally.

The dancer should not handle a blood blister in this manner but should treat it by applying a doughnut and allowing the blister to reabsorb by itself. The reason for extreme care in cases of blood blisters is their predisposition to infection when additionally irritated.

If any blister has been torn, it is desirable to cleanse the area thoroughly with an antiseptic such as Merthiolate and then pack it with a salve antiseptic such as zinc oxide. The skin flap is placed over the salve packing and a doughnut applied around its perimeter. When handled in this manner, the torn blister usually will not become contaminated, because the salve provides protection from further infection and injury. In 2 or 3 days the skin can be cut away and the salve removed, allowing the new tendon skin to be toughened (Fig. 11-7).

CORNS

Corns are the result of abnormal pressure from improperly fitting shoes. They are of two types: hard corns (Calvus durum) and soft corns (Calvus mole). In both cases the pressures that come from the shoe cause the top tissue layer to be pressed inward, causing a corn-shaped growth to occur. Because it presses on nerve endings and causes inflammation, the corn can be extremely painful and handicapping. The hard corn is associated with hammer toe because of the skin pressure of the toe against the top of the shoe. The soft corn is less serious than the hard corn and is usually found

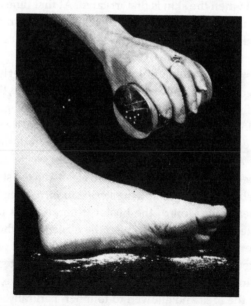

Fig. 11-7. Talcum powder helps eliminate friction.

between the fourth and fifth toes. Painful hard corns must be referred to a specialist. However, the soft corn may be managed by some of the more common commercial medications on the market. Eliminating the basic cause often gives immediate relief. For example, flattening the clawed or hammer toe with a piece of tape may relieve the pain of the hard corn (Fig. 11-3), and the soft corn can be relieved by separating the toes with lamb's wool or cotton (Fig. 11-8).

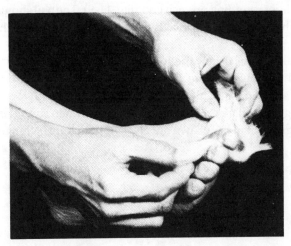

Fig. 11-8. Lamb's wool can often relieve the pain of a soft corn.

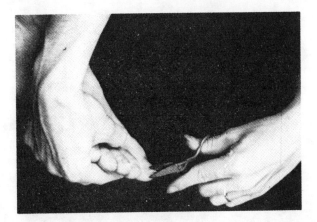

Fig. 11-9. Toenails should be trimmed straight across with a slight rounding on each end.

INGROWN TOENAIL

The ingrown toenail, like other foot conditions, can be the result of abnormal pressure from too short or too narrow shoes. Dancing on pointe may also cause this problem. Whatever the cause, the side edge of the toenail grows into the soft tissue of the skin, bringing about severe irritation and often infection. The ingrown toenail can be an extremely disabling condition and must be avoided. Avoidance is best accomplished by proper footwear and proper trimming of the toenails. The toenail should always be trimmed straight across with a slight rounding on each end (Fig. 11-9). The nail should never be rounded to the extent that it contacts the skin on either side of the nail bed.

If an ingrown toenail does occur, the foot should be soaked in 110°F water 2 or 3 times daily, followed by the application of a thin wisp of cotton under the edge of the affected nail. This approach lifts the nail slightly from the nail bed, providing immediate relief from pain. This regimen should be continued until the ingrown nail has grown out and symptoms are no longer present.

12

Strains

As discussed earlier, the abnormal pull of the musculotendinous unit is one of the dancer's most pressing problems. Fatigue, faulty body alignment, or improper dance technique can cause an overstretching or tearing of muscle fibers. The dancer usually experiences fatigue, spasm, and then the pain of stretching or tearing of the muscle. The onset of a strain can be prevented by stopping the activity at the point of fatigue. However, the sense of fatigue is often ignored with the mistaken idea that for progress to occur there must be discomfort in the body. This mistaken concept may eventually produce a chronic pathological condition, incurring the risk of ruining a successful career.

Another mistaken idea that many dancers have is that a part should be only stretched without the important backup program of muscle strengthening. Overstretching the musculoskeletal unit often produces a lack of awareness of when a muscle has been lengthened too far. Stretching and full range of movement are necessary for success in dance; however, this should never be indulged in to the detriment of adequate muscle tone in a particular part.

ACUTE STRAINS

The acute strain (Table 10), like the contusion, is divided into first-, second-, and third-degree intensity. However, in many cases it is advisable that strains be treated as if they were one degree greater in intensity than they appear to be, because it is difficult to categorize an injury as to its exact degree of intensity. There is a wide disparity in each degree of injury intensity;

175

Table 10. Acute strain management

Degree of injury	Basic signs	Treatment program				
		Management phase	Physical therapy	Dosage	Reconditioning	Dosage
First degree	Mild pull or stretch of musculotendinous unit causing spasm and sometimes pain and tenderness	Step 1: immediate care	1. Apply cold and pressure 2. Ice massage if spasm is suspected	24 hr Daily	1. Gradual stretch following ice massage	Daily
Second degree	Moderate stretch and tear of portions of musculotendinous unit causing extreme spasm, point tenderness, loss of function, swelling, and discoloration	Step 1: immediate care	1. Apply cold and pressure; 20 min on, 20 min off 2. Elevation 3. Wear elastic wrap 4. Medication	24–48 hr 24–48 hr As prescribed	1. Avoid exercise and stretch of part 2. General sustained exercise	Daily
		Step 2: second or third day	1. Gradual heating of part if hemorrhage has stopped; use superficial devices (soaks and pads at 100° F, whirlpool not to exceed 90° F for 10 min), contrast bath 2. Massage above and below injury	Twice daily 5 min twice daily	1. Avoid exercise and stretch of part 2. Continue general sustained exercise	Twice daily
		Step 3: third or fourth day	1. Continue superficial heat (soaks at 110° F, whirlpool at 102° F)	15 min three times daily	1. Avoid forced stretching of part 2. Start exercising part (ROM)	Daily

Degree	Step	Treatment	Frequency		Frequency
	Step 4: fourth or fifth day	2. Massage above and below injury	5 min three times daily	3. Continue general sustained exercise of entire body	Twice daily
		3. Contrast bath	Twice daily		
		4. Analgesic balm	When active		
		5. Elastic wrap	When active		
		1. Superficial heat	20 min three times daily	1. Begin easy stretch of part (if pain free)	Daily
		2. Massage	Three times daily	2. Start program of PRE (progressive resistance exercise)	Twice daily
		3. Contrast bath	Twice daily	3. Continue program of general sustained exercise	Twice daily
		4. Deep heat, if available	As prescribed		
		5. Analgesic balm or liniment	Symptomatic		
		6. Ice massage with gradual stretch	Daily		
		7. Elastic wrap	When active		
	Step 5	1. Therapy program is continued until dancer is symptom free	Three times daily	1. Continue until symptom free	Three times daily
Third degree	Step 1: immediate care	Severe muscle stretch causing extensive tissue tearing, rupture, or pulling away from bone			
		1. Refer to physician for x-ray examination and medication		1. Rest	48-72 hr
		2. Apply cold and pressure; 20 min on, 20 min off	48-72 hr		
		3. Elevation of part	48-72 hr		
		4. Elastic wrap			
	Step 2: third or fourth day	1. Superficial heat	10 min twice daily	1. Avoid exercising and stretching part	
		2. Contrast bath	Twice daily		

Continued.

Table 10. Acute strain management—cont'd.

Degree of injury	Basic signs	Management phase	Treatment program			
			Physical therapy	Dosage	Reconditioning	Dosage
		Step 3: fourth or fifth day	3. Massage above and below injury	5 min twice daily	2. Start general sustained exercise	Daily
			4. Elastic wrap			
			1. Superficial heat	Three times daily	1. Avoid exercising and stretching part	
			2. Contrast bath	Three times daily	2. General sustained exercise	Twice daily
			3. Massage above and below injury	Three times daily		
			4. Analgesic balm or liniment	When active		
			5. Elastic wrap			
		Step 4: fifth or sixth and following days	1. Superficial heat	20 min three times daily	1. Begin easy stretching of part if pain free	Daily
			2. Contrast bath	Three times daily	2. Start PRE	Twice daily
			3. Massage	5 min three times daily	3. Continue general sustained exercise	Twice daily
			4. Deep heat	As prescribed		
			5. Analgesic balm or liniment	When active		
			6. Elastic wrap			
		Step 5	1. Therapy program is continued until dancer is symptom free	Three times daily	1. Continue until symptom free	Three times daily

therefore, if a dancer is in doubt about the degree of an injury, it should be treated as if it were more severe than the symptoms indictate.

The symptoms of a first-degree strain can range from a very slight twinge in a muscle and soreness following activity to a local spasm with some muscle weakness. There may even be some point tenderness in the area. Often the dancer is not aware that a mild strain has occurred and will not realize it until the next day when soreness is present. Most of the discomfort of the first-degree sprain is due to muscle spasm and not to the tearing of muscle fibers. Therefore, cold is applied to the area for up to 24 hours either by ice pack or by ice massage. If this is followed by a gradual stretch, much of the pain and discomfort can be eliminated. If soreness persists after stretching, then a procedure of warm water soaks or warm (not to exceed 90°F) whirlpool treatment may be initiated. A gradual stretching regimen should be continued until soreness has completely subsided. In cases where soreness persists for more than 2 days, it is suggested that an elastic wrap be worn around the part to provide a mild external massage agent and at the same time provide some support to the injured muscle.

As in all cases of strain, the second-degree strain is caused by a traumatic stretch of the musculotendinous unit that results in pain, a burning sensation, and a loss of function for a short period. Spasm as well as hemorrhaging and swelling is usually associated with this problem. Swelling can be effectively controlled by a cold compress and elevation of the part immediately following the injury. Ideally, if a physican is immediately available, the dancer with a second-degree strain may profit from medications that might consist of muscle relaxants and/or enzymes. If the loss of function lasts for more than a half an hour following proper immediate care, referral to a physician is routine. To most effectively assist nature in resolving the inflammatory process, it is suggested that the dancer apply cold compresses and elevate the part for at least 24 to 48 hours, depending on how quickly discomfort is overcome and function returns. At no time should the dancer attempt to stretch out this condition, because torn tissue is always associated with the second-degree strain.

When the immediate phase of this injury has been resolved and hemorrhage appears to be under control, a gradual warming process can begin first by whirlpool, if available, with a temperature of 90°F for approximately 10 minutes or a heating pad set at warm (not hot) for approximately 20 minutes. An elastic wrap should be worn around the part to provide continual pressure and soft-tissue support, particularly when the dancer engages in physical activity. The dancer should gradually increase the temperature of the whirlpool or immersion baths over 4 or 5 days until the maximum is reached. The dancer should begin a general exercise or activities program that excludes the affected part. Specific exercise of the affected part should start when there is no discomfort with movement. At no time should the dancer attempt to stretch the moderate strain if pain is present. A program of specific therapeutic exercises can be instituted along with flexibility exercises when the injury is symptom-free.

The third-degree strain is the most severe of all strains, and when it is incurred the dancer must be immediately referred to a physican for treatment. Determination of this degree of injury, as well as all other degrees, is best made by how much function is lost in the injured part. Typically the dancer will complain of a sudden snap or tear and perhaps a sudden burning sensation in the affected part along with muscle spasm, point tenderness, and inability to fully contract the muscle. If the strain was sustained at the muscle origin, or its insertion, the dancer should suspect the possibility of the muscle having been torn away from the bone. If the injury occurs to the soft belly portion of the muscle, the possibility of muscle rupture should be entertained. In any case, if an avulsion fracture is suspected, the severe strain demands immediate referral to a physican for X-ray examination, and medication. If a muscle rupture or avulsion fracture occurs, surgical repair must be performed as soon as possible for the best results. If the strain is uncomplicated, immediate care consisting of cold, pressure, and evaluation is carried out for as long as 72 hours, whereas gradual heating is not usually begun for about 3 or 4 days after the initial injury has occurred.

After the immediate care phase, the dancer should engage in a general exercise program while avoiding movements that may aggravate the injury. As indicated earlier, the generalized exercise program encourages the healing process, and there should be a decrease in the amount of scar tissue at the strain site. An elastic wrap should be kept on the affected part while the dancer is active or until the part is symptom-free. Specific progressive exercise is not given to the affected part until about 5 days to a week following the initial injury episode, at which time a gradual program of strengthening and flexibility is started. The dancer should not be in too much of a hurry to return to full activity. Attempting to force an injury to heal before nature has intended or engaging in activity before the injury has become resolved often produces a subacute or chronic condition. This is particularly true when there has been an overstretching of a tendon. A dancer should allow the body to heal the injury in its own time. To be in too much of a hurry causes more scarring than usual, increases the susceptibility to a recurrence of the same injury, and produces a chronic problem.

Cramps or muscle spasms

Muscle spasms have been discussed throughout this book as being associated with any compression or stretching of soft tissue. Although not always obvious to the dancer, the muscle cramp is also a muscle spasm. However, the cramp may be considered a sudden violent and involuntary contraction of the muscle that is immediately painful. Muscle cramping can be either *clonic* or *tonic*. The clonic cramp is identified by intermittent contraction and relaxation of the muscle, pulsating almost like a heart beat, whereas the tonic type is a steady or constant contraction of a particular muscle. The direct cause of the cramp is difficult to pinpoint, but fatigue, fluid and mineral depletion through excessive perspiration, and the breaking down of reciprocal muscle coordination are major causative factors. Sometimes the cramp occurs during some activity, and at other times it occurs when the dancer is at rest or asleep.

When a cramp occurs, the dancer should never attempt to dance through the problem but should stop immediately and attempt to reduce the cramp. Initially a cramp should not be massaged but should be grasped firmly, with constant pressure applied until it subsides. When the cramp has melted away, a gradual stretch can be applied to the area, followed by a more vigorous stretch when the cramp is completely under control. After stretching, the cramp can be treated by application of superficial heat. If the dancer has cramps daily in different areas of the body, referral to a physican is necessary. The physican may prescribe an electrolyte supplementation as a possible approach to alleviating the problem.

Foot and ankle strain

Strains about the foot are common in dance and occur often to the toes, the arch, or the ankle region. Foot and ankle strains often come from dancing on very hard unyielding surfaces. The toe most often strained is the great toe, which is primarily used in propelling the dancer in leaps and landings. Often associated with foot and ankle strain is faulty foot alignment such as seen in dancers with extremely high or low longitudinal arches. Malalignment affecting the entire foot and leading to strain often stems from a forced turn-out by the dancer that abducts the forefoot upon the midfoot. Foot varus may also occur from a short leg, subsequently resulting in foot muscle imbalance.

Plantar fascia strain. The plantar fascial strain is prevalent among dancers and, like toe problems, occurs mainly from jumping and landing movements. Continuous straining leads to the fallen arch. Because of the site and nature of the strain, it readily becomes a chronic problem of fasciitis.[20]

Hot water soaks or whirlpool hydromassage treatment several times a day coupled with strapping support for the longitudinal arch is essential for remediation. Routing arch exercises along with Achilles tendon stretching are essential treatment procedures.

Technique A: simple arch strapping with pad (Fig. 12-1, A). The dancer with mild pain and general discomfort in the various foot tendons can find relief by applying two or three strips of 1½-inch linen-backed tape or two strips of 2-inch elastic tape around the arch. However, a more substantial technique is to incorporate a sponge rubber pad along the longitudinal arch area, combining it with circles of tape. The pad is made of ¼-inch sponge rubber cut to the shape of the individual arch.

Technique B: arch X strapping (Fig. 12-1, B). This technique is designed to provide some support for the longitudinal arch and is particularly valuable in cases of arch strain or the beginning of a fallen arch. The procedure is to first apply a 1-inch circle of tape around the ball of the foot to act as an anchor for

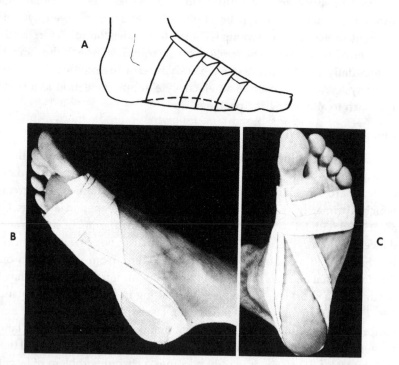

Fig. 12-1. Arch support techniques. **A,** Simple arch strapping with pad. **B,** Arch X strapping. **C,** Single cross arch strapping.

the major support tape. The tape starts from the metatarsophalangeal joint of the great toe, crosses the center of the arch, goes around the heel, and goes back across the center of the arch, ending at the metatarsophalangeal joint on the little toe side. This procedure is repeated once more and is then locked in place by circles of tape placed around the ball and arch. If possible, the technique should be finished with 2-inch elastic tape.

Technique C: single or double cross arch strapping (Fig. 12-1, C). This technique is designed for the more severely strained arch and also can be used for realigning a twisted forefoot. As in technique B, the circle of tape is placed around the metatarsophalangeal joint loosely to act as an anchor for the arch tape strips. Starting on either side of the foot, a strip of 1-inch tape is run from the metatarsophalangeal joint straight along the side of the foot and around the heel, crossing the center of the arch and ending at the point where the tape began. The technique is repeated on the other side of the foot. Both procedures are repeated again until two strips of tape have been applied to each side of the foot.

Achilles tendon strain. Strain of the Achilles tendon is also frequent in dance and is caused by a sudden overstretching of the Achilles tendon due to a forcible pushing of the foot against the floor, usually resulting from leaping and stage running ball-to-heel instead of heel-to-ball. Also, the dancer who has a tendon narrower than 3/8 inch has a tendency toward straining.[21] In this situation, the Achilles tendon is stretched and then contracts suddenly, which causes a tissue tear. This problem should be immediately treated and protected against another injury, because the Achilles tendon rapidly tends to develop a chronic condition following one or more acute strain episodes.

Leg strain

Hamstring strain. Hamstring strains have a high incidence in most physically active persons who use their legs extensively. The reason for this high incidence is difficult to determine. In dance the hamstring group is often extensively stretched without a protective strengthening program (Fig. 12-2). An imbalance in the strength of the quadricepsmuscle in front of the thigh and the hamstring group in back of the thigh predisposes the hamstring to spasm, fatigue, and subsequent strain. Susceptibility to hamstring strain is also prevalent in those persons who have a strength difference of more than 10% between the left and right hamstring group and those in whom a hamstring group has 50% less strength than the opposing quadriceps muscle group.

When it comes to conditioning and injury prevention, one must consider

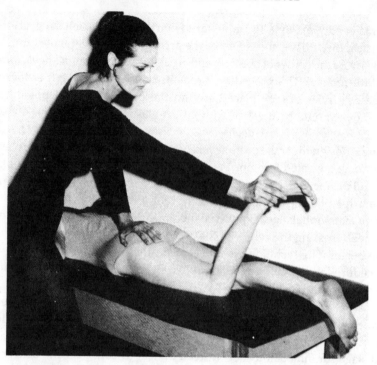

Fig. 12-2. Strengthening the hamstring muscles.

the hamstrings as the most neglected muscle group in the body. Therefore, the dancer should include leg flexion and hip extension movements (for example, passé to attitude to arabesque) in the conditioning program whenever possible. The hamstring strain is often obvious to the dancer before it occurs. Fatigue is the first and most obvious sign; it is followed by spasm and then the actual stretching and tearing of muscle tissue. If the hamstring area feels tired or "dead," the dancer should avoid all stretching and dance activities that may overly stress this area and should immediately engage in a gradual strengthening program.

Treatment of the hamstring strain is in keeping with care of any typical strain. However, the dancer should be encouraged to engage in a general movement program as soon as possible. It is desirable that the general exercise program consist of many locomotor activities that do not overly fatigue or stretch the hamstring muscles. For protection the dancer should wear an elastic wrap around the thigh. The elastic wrap provides a mild support to the muscles and helps prevent overstretching and aggravation of the area. If the dancer must engage in vigorous activity even though the hamstring strain has not completely recovered, a tape support can be utilized.

Hamstring strapping (Fig. 12-3). Both the hamstring and the quadriceps muscle groups can be protected by X strapping. This technique is designed to support muscles against gravity and to provide external soft compression. The materials for the hamstring X technique can be either 1- or 2-inch linen tape or, ideally, 2- or 3-inch elastic tape. The hamstring technique is started by a strip of tape between 6 and 9 inches long on each side of the thigh. With the lower leg slightly bent to relax the hamstring muscles, the tape is crisscrossed starting just above the bend of the knee and working upward to the base of the buttock. When the crisscrossing has been completed strips of tape are applied on both sides of the thigh to hold the X's in place. Finally, elastic wrap is applied to the thigh to prevent the tape from becoming loose during activity.

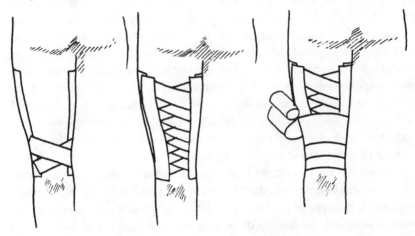

Fig. 12-3. Hamstring X strapping.

Anterior thigh strain. In general, strain to the rectus femoris muscle is relatively rare. However, of those strains that do occur, more occur to the female dancer. The reason for this may be the difference in the line of muscle pull resulting from the female's slightly wider pelvis. Unlike the hamstring strain, which often occurs from a sudden abnormal stretch, the quadriceps strain occurs primarily from a static muscle contraction. For example, the dancer places the quadriceps muscle in stretch by bending the knee about 40 degrees and then attempts to hold this position, exerting a stress on the full length of the muscle. Like the hamstring strain, the quadriceps strain can be protected from repeated trauma by the application of a tape or elastic wrap support. It should also be noted that jumping, landing, and locking the knees suddenly causes a common dance problem in which the patellar tendon is repeatedly pulled, resulting in patellar tendinitis. Because dancers seldom run with legs facing straight ahead the sartorius muscle has a higher incidence of injury to the anterior thigh region than the quadriceps group. Additional discussion of the quadriceps strain will be presented in the section on chronic strains.

Groin strain

Crossing the hip joint are a great many muscles and tendons that allow the thigh full mobility. The dancer places great demands on the full mobility of the hip, frequently overstretching the muscles and supportive tissue in that area. The groin, which is the region lying between the thigh and the abdomen, is one of the most often strained areas in dance. The muscles in the area of the groin primarily allow the dancer to flex, adduct, and inwardly rotate the thigh. These actions are produced by the iliopsoas, the rectus femoris, and the adductor muscle groups and the intrinsic internal rotators. Like many other muscles and groups of muscles that are susceptible to strain, there is often an imbalance between agonist and antagonist groin muscles, one overpowering the other. The stronger and tighter muscles are least able to withstand a sudden stretch and the weaker muscles are more susceptible to fatigue. In the groin region, the hip flexors overpower the extenders, abductors, adductors, and external rotators. It is necessary, therefore, that a balance of strength and flexibility be sought.

Because of the complexity of the muscles in the hip region, it is important for the dancer to know whether the strain is accessible to topical therapy or whether it is deep, requiring more definitive professional care. The less serious strain can be dealt with by cold and superficial heat, but the deep strain is not readily amenable to any physical therapy approach and is usually self-limiting. The self-limiting injury is one in which therapy does little good.

To determine the seriousness of a groin strain it is advisable that a functional test be given. The first test is for the rectus femoris, the only two-joint muscle of the quadriceps group (Fig. 12-4). This relatively superficial muscle, besides extending the knee, crosses the hip joint and assists the dancer in flexing the thigh or bending the trunk forward. To test this muscle, the dancer sits on a table with both legs hanging over the end. While the dancer extends the affected leg, gradual resistance is applied until it is fully extended. This application of resistance puts stress specifically on the rectus femoris muscle; if a strain is present, pain will be felt in the groin area. A second test for a fairly superficial muscle group is the thigh adductor test (Fig. 12-5). In this test the dancer lies on a table with the affected leg abducted as wide as possible. The leg is then pulled to the midline position against

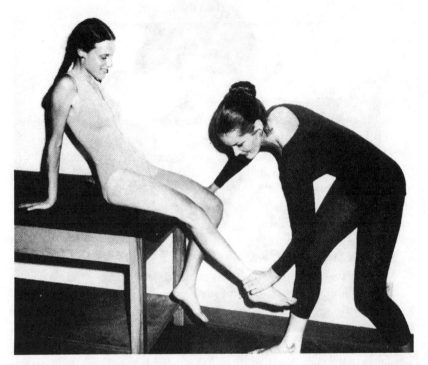

Fig. 12-4. Leg extension against resistance to test for strain of rectus femoris muscle.

resistance. If pain is felt on this movement, it is assumed that one of the adductor muscles is strained.

The third test, which is designed to reflect strain in the deep iliopsoas muscle of the hip, requires the dancer to sit on the edge of a table with both legs hanging over the end. The dancer then lifts the affected thigh upward against a resistance. A strain of the iliopsoas would be identified by a deep pain in the groin area. Without the full function of the iliopsoas, the dancer is unable to efficiently maintain an upright posture and to move the thigh effectively. The treatment of groin strain should be conservative, including avoidance of physical activity as long as possible and engaging in such physical therapy as whirlpool, hot packs, and, in the case of deeper injuries, diathermy and ultrasound therapy. If exercise must be engaged in, the dancer should wear a groin support wrap to decrease the possibilities of overstretching.

Groin wrap (Fig. 12-6). The groin wrap is a spica bandage applied in a specific manner to help the dancer decrease the chances of reinjury. A 4- or

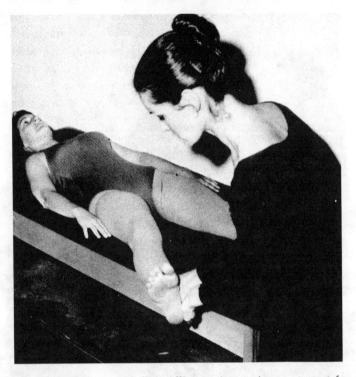

Fig. 12-5. Pressing thigh toward the midline against resistance to test for strain of the adductor muscles.

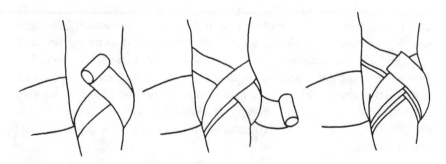

Fig. 12-6. Groin wrap.

6-inch elastic wrap is used. The dancer stands with the affected thigh turned inward. The wrap is started at the upper end of the inner side of the thigh, carried to the inside, and then wrapped around the outside and over the crest of the ilium in front of the abdomen. It is then carried around the back, and the same pattern is retraced until all the material is applied. If additional support is needed, a pad should be placed on the strained site for additional compression. To ensure greater stability, elastic tape could also be applied by tracing the pattern of the wrap.

Snapping hip

Dancers commonly complain of a snap occurring in the hip, especially when he or she stands in a relaxed posture with body weight sagging onto one hip (Fig. 12-7), which may lead to a snapping hip. The snapping is caused by the greater trochanter of the femur moving outward, creating a popping sound. In analysis of the problem it is speculated that balancing on one foot produces a submaximal contraction of the abductor muscles, which serve to stabilize the pelvis in relation to the thigh, primarily the gluteus medius and tensor fasciae latae muscles. Another occasion on which the snapping hip is pronounced is when the grand ronde de jambe technique is performed. Specifically, as the leg is moved down toward the floor a snap occurs. In their study, Jacobs and Young[13] found that a slow ronde de jambe en l'air is a major cause of snapping hip. In this technique the dancer starts with the hip flexed, and the thigh in a sagittal plane moves from abduction in a frontal plane, hip laterally rotated and the knee fully extended or performing a slow grand battement, which is hip flexion in the sagittal plane. In these techniques, the connective tissue and tendons crossing the hip joint of the support leg tend to give way. The iliofemoral ligament (Y ligament) may also produce the snapping or clicking sound as it moves over the femoral head during hip flexion or abduction in the sagittal and frontal planes, respectively (Fig. 12-8). Jacobs and Young found that dancers with snapping hips have a narrower hip, greater range of hip abduction, and less lateral rotation than a comparable group of dancers who do not have the problem of snapping hip. Although pain is seldom associated with the snapping hip, degeneration of the greater trochanter has been suggested as a possible outcome when the snapping hip is experienced over a long period. Two procedures have been found to assist in remediation of this problem: strengthening the abductor muscle of the hip (see Fig. 6-19), and stretching the tensor fasciae latae muscle (see Fig. 6-13).

Back and neck strain

The spine is an area of the body that is extremely vulnerable to strain in dance. Exceeding the individual limits of the back often results in muscular

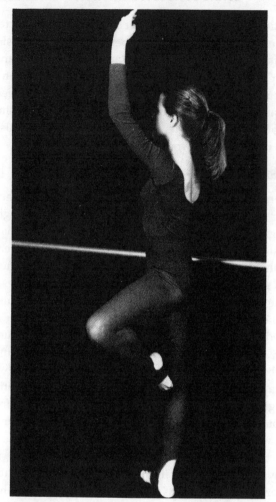

Fig. 12-7. Sagging onto the hip on the support side may lead to a snapping hip.

strain and, more seriously, in a sprain. The spine allows a great variety of movements. For example, flexion is allowed in the neck, or cervical, region and the upper thoracic, lumbar, and lumbosacral regions. Hyperextension of the back is mainly prevented in the thoracic vertebrae by the protruding spinal processes. Side bending, or lateral flexion, occurs in the cervical area and in a somewhat limited degree in the lumbar area. Rotation occurs freely in the neck as a result of the lack of heavy, bony, interlocking articular processes of the cervical vertebrae.

Many factors make the back and neck prone to injury. The most common of these factors are due to the great diversity in how backs are anatomically formed. Posture, body alignment, and the dancer's attempt to exceed the

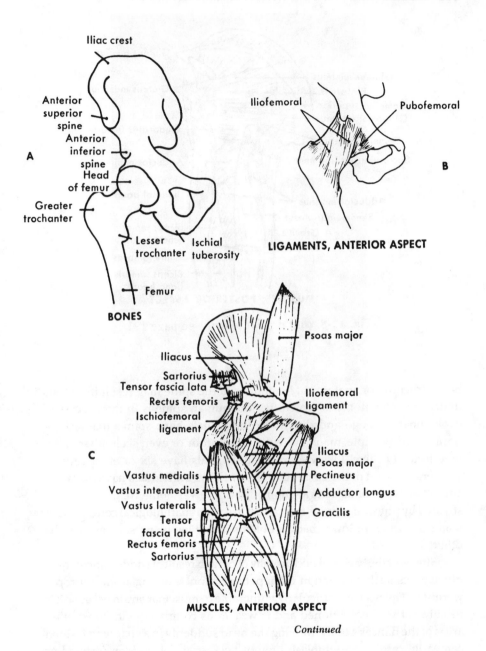

BONES

Iliac crest

Anterior superior spine

Anterior inferior spine

Head of femur

Greater trochanter

Lesser trochanter

Ischial tuberosity

Femur

A

LIGAMENTS, ANTERIOR ASPECT

Iliofemoral

Pubofemoral

B

MUSCLES, ANTERIOR ASPECT

Psoas major

Iliacus

Sartorius

Tensor fascia lata

Rectus femoris

Ischiofemoral ligament

Iliofemoral ligament

Vastus medialis

Vastus intermedius

Vastus lateralis

Tensor fascia lata

Rectus femoris

Sartorius

Iliacus

Psoas major

Pectineus

Adductor longus

Gracilis

C

Continued

Fig. 12-8. Hip anatomy. **A,** Bone structure. **B,** Ligaments, anterior aspect. **C,**Muscles, anterior aspect. **D,** Muscles, posterior aspect. (**A, C,** and **D** from Klafs, C. E., and Arnheim, D.D.: Modern principles of athletic training, ed. 4, St. Louis, 1977, The C.V. Mosby Co.)

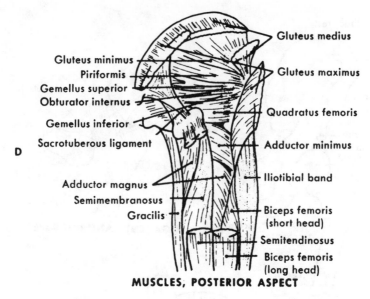

Gluteus medius

Gluteus minimus
Piriformis
Gemellus superior
Obturator internus

Gluteus maximus

Quadratus femoris

Gemellus inferior

Sacrotuberous ligament

Adductor minimus

D

Iliotibial band

Adductor magnus
Semimembranosus
Gracilis

Biceps femoris
(short head)

Semitendinosus

Biceps femoris
(long head)

MUSCLES, POSTERIOR ASPECT

Fig. 12-8, cont'd.   For legend see page 191.

basic structural or anatomical limitations of the spine may result in serious injury. It is commonly accepted that the human spine is in the process of evolutionary change and that many individuals have spines that are abnormal. For example, many individuals have four or even six lumbar vertebrae instead of five. Likewise many individuals have six or eight cervical vertebrae instead of the customary seven. Some individuals have extra ribs and other types of structural anomalies of the vertebrae that, when overstressed by physical activity, may result in serious pathological conditions. A major precursor of lower back problems is one leg being shorter than the other.

Strains of the back and neck usually occur as a result of sudden uncommon movements such as rotation or hyperextension resulting from improper warm-up. The neck is particularly vulnerable to muscular strain because it is usually not well conditioned and is weaker as compared with most other areas of the dancer's body. Moving the head suddenly in a snapping fashion can easily result in a whiplash type of neck strain. A sudden forward or backward movement of the trunk can produce spasm strain with severe handicapping pain. Susceptibility to low back strain is increased by the postural problem of lordosis with its associated tight lower back and weak abdominal musculature. The male dancer is particularly susceptible to back strains when he is executing a lift.

Sudden acute injury to the neck and back again should be treated as any typical strain. However, because of the back's propensity to muscle spasm, rather than to tearing of muscle tissue, the practice of ice massage combined with a gradual stretch often relieves the symptoms almost instantaneously. This is particularly true in the cervical, upper back, and lumbar regions. Dancers with injuries to the back and neck that do not respond to palliative treatment within a week should be routinely referred to a physician.

Arm and shoulder strain

In dancers the incidence of arm strain is not as high as the incidence of strain of the lower limbs. There are occasions, however, when the dancer strains muscles in the arm or shoulder because of a fall on an outstretched arm, a sudden twist, or the lifting of a heavy load. The shoulder's basic design is for full mobility; hence, it is seldom strained in dance except in a situation where there is extreme rotation, such as falling on the arm in an awkward position or lifting a partner when off balance. This causes strain of the small intrinsic muscles of the shoulder that cause inward and outward rotation. The dancer who is unable to internally or externally rotate the shoulder without pain or who is unable to raise the arm out to the side may be considered to have strained the deeper muscles of the shoulder such as the rotator cuff. Topical therapy to the shoulder is not usually effective, but moist heat does have some palliative effect in relaxation of the overly tense muscles. Often the therapy of choice in injuries to the shoulder is ultrasound or diathermy. The most important concern in managing a strained shoulder is to overcome the problem of immobility, which often results in muscle contractures together with a severe loss of movement. It is important that the dancer try to maintain a normal range of shoulder movement without aggravating the condition. This means that in the early stages of injury, rotation of the shoulder should be maintained by nongravity-type exercises. For example, the affected arm is rotated while it is allowed to hang down in a relaxed manner. When the dancer is pain free and able to initiate a regular exercise program, the concern should be full-range activities in the upright posture. Progressive resistance exercises of the shoulder should not be initiated until the dancer can easily execute free shoulder movements while standing in the upright posture.

A relatively common problem among dancers is sciatica, or sciatic nerve syndrome. The sciatic nerve is the largest nerve in the body, arising from the sacral nerve plexus on either side of the body, passing from the pelvis through the greater sciatic foramen, or notch, and down the back of the thigh, dividing into smaller nerves, and ending in the region of the foot. The cause of sciatica is compression of the sciatic nerve or its roots. The common cause in dancers is from pressure on the nerve by the outward rotator muscles, which are characteristically overly tight in comparison to the inward rotators. Sciatica may be characterized by a sharp, shooting pain running down the back of the thigh and/or leg that is intensified by movement. There may also be numbness and a tingling sensation. Rest, combined with various forms of physical therapy, is typical treatment. Exercise including stretching and increasing the strength of the internal rotators may give relief.

The elbow and wrist have a lower incidence of injury in dance than does the shoulder. Normally the elbow is strong and can withstand the rigors placed on it; in contrast, the wrist is more vulnerable to injury, mainly in attempting to brace the body in a fall. As in reconditioning of the shoulder, one should first be concerned with maintaining the range of movement in the elbow. However, the elbow must never be forced to regain its flexibility but should be allowed to do so gradually. This is because the injured elbow tends to rapidly develop contractures and scar tissue when placed in a forced program of reconditioning. The wrist injury, specifically the sprain, is discussed in Chapter 13.

CHRONIC STRAINS

The chronic strain (Table 11) comes about from many acute episodes that can result in a variety of conditions such as myositis, fascitis, tendinitis, tenosynovitis, or bursitis, depending on the particular injury site and body tissue involved. As with other chronic conditions, the chronic strain represents a constantly irritated area that has developed an inflammation within the tissues that the body is unable to overcome. Dancers, because of their desire for perfection and their fear that if they miss a class or practice session their technique will deteriorate, often place themselves in a situation where a chronic strain is inevitable. In most cases, if the acute single strain episode were properly cared for, the chronic problem would not occur.

Fallen arch

The fallen arch is attributed to the chronically stretched tendons and ligaments of the foot. Once fallen, the arch cannot be restored. Consequently, preventing the initial problem or preventing further falling is of major concern to the dancer. To prevent the arch from dropping, a daily routine of foot exercises should be undertaken, along with avoidance of activities that put a great deal of abnormal strain on the foot, such as dancing on hard,

Table 11. Chronic strain management

Common conditions	Basic signs	Treatment program					
		Management phase	Physical therapy	Dosage	Reconditioning	Dosage
Simple muscle soreness	Mild to moderate muscle tenderness on palpation and movement	Symptomatic	1. Ice massage followed by gradual stretch	Two to three times daily	1. Gradual stretching	Two to three times daily
Tendinitis, tenosynovitis, myositis, fasciitis, and bursitis	Continuous low-grade inflammation with pain on movement, local weakness with restriction on muscle stretching, and point tenderness	Symptomatic	1. Superficial heat	Three times daily	1. Rest	
			2. Ice massage after stretch	Two to three times daily	2. Gradual stretching	Two to three times daily
			3. Deep heat	As prescribed		
			4. Anti-inflammatory drugs	As prescribed		

nonresilient surfaces. Sore arches will benefit from therapy procedures such as hot water soaks at 110°F several times daily combined with supportive taping.

Achilles tendinitis

The Achilles tendon is highly susceptible to strain. Repeated strain to this area results in a condition known as tendinitis, in which the tendon becomes chronically inflamed. Because the Achilles tendon is involved in almost all foot movement, it is difficult to prevent further irritation once an injury has been incurred. Another problem associated with the overstretching of the Achilles tendon is an inflammation of the bursa that is present where the Achilles tendon joins the calcaneus. This bursa can also be irritated by the constant pressure of dance shoes, producing symptoms similar to those of the strained Achilles tendon.

The dancer with these problems should make every effort to avoid irritating activity and to shorten the Achilles tendon by raising the heel with a customized pad. When street shoes are worn, a ¼-inch sponge rubber pad placed under each heel will help alleviate some of the irritation. If dancing must be undertaken, Achilles tendon strapping should be applied.

Achilles tendon strapping (Fig. 12-9). The technique for Achilles tendon strapping uses 2- or 3-inch elastic tape and 1-inch linen tape. The foot should be relaxed completely, and two 1-inch anchor strips applied around the ball of the foot and lower leg approximately 4 to 5 inches above the malleolus (ankle bone). One strip of elastic tape is then placed starting at the ball of the foot, stretched across the bottom of the foot and up the back of the heel, and joined to the anchor strip around the leg. This first elastic tape strip should be stretched firmly but not to the full extent of the tape. A second strip is applied over the first but is cut approximately 4 inches longer. The upper end of the second strip is cut and split lengthwise, with each separate strip wrapped around the lower leg, forming a lock. This technique is completed with two or three anchor strips wrapped around the foot and the lower leg. Achilles tendon strapping still allows the dancer to move but prevents the Achilles tendon from being overstretched.

Shin splints

Shin splints is one of the most common problems that plague dancers and is usually caused by repetitive use of the foot flexors on hard surfaces.[25] It is characterized by leg pain and irritation, and the legs become increasingly more tender and sore after vigorous activity has ceased. The specific site of shin splints is often vague but is commonly thought to be the posterior or

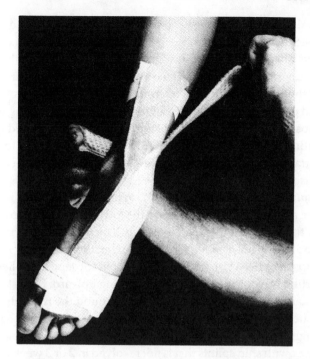

Fig. 12-9. Achilles tendon strapping.

anterior tibial muscles or the interossei muscles between the tibia and fibula. It is characterized by a dull ache in the lower shin area. This condition most often occurs during the very early conditioning period of new classes, indicating inadequate fitness, and again toward the end of classes, which would indicate fatigue. Dancers who have abnormally externally rotated their lower extremities in the turn-out, who have performed duck-footed running, or who have pronated feet are highly susceptible to shin splints. Other factors that seem to increase the incidence of this problem. Because of the great diversity of possible causes, one can deduce that shin splints are caused mainly by a lack of reciprocal coordination between opposing muscles of the lower leg resulting from one muscle pulling against another. The cause of shin splints may be present alone or in combination with two or even three other conditions; therefore, it is difficult to pinpoint the exact reason why a dancer develops this problem. Once dancers contract skin splints, susceptibility is greater in the future.

The treatment of shin splints is usually symptomatic, the most beneficial approach being the continual application of superficial heat over a long period. Whirlpool at 102°F or hot water soaks at 110°F and the application of analgesic balm packs have been found to be the most effective treatment procedures. Such physical therapy modalities as diathermy and ultrasound therapy have not proved to be any more beneficial to the dancer than the less expensive superficial approach. Along with the superficial heat treatment, the dancer should engage in a stretch routine that includes stretching of the anterior and posterior muscles both before and after activity (Figs. 6-1 and 6-2). Also, those dancers who have a history of shin splints should make this stretch routine a preventive procedure. In order for a dancer to continue activity, a strapping technique should be used that will alleviate some of the pain and discomfort.

Shin splints strapping (Fig. 12-10). While the dancer is in a seated position, the affected leg is bent, causing the lower leg muscles to be relaxed and soft to the touch. In this leg position a 1-inch by 2-inch strip of foam rubber or adhesive felt is applied directly over the sore area. A series of circular strips of either 1½-inch linen or 2-inch lastic tape is applied around the leg, starting below the irritation and working upward. Each strip of tape should be started from the back and brought around the front, drawing the muscle tissue to the bone. It is also advantageous to apply either the the figure-of-eight or the arch X strapping around the longitudinal arch of the foot. A dancer with shin splints that is not resolved in 2 or 3 weeks should be automatically referred to a physician because of the possibility of stress fracture in this area.

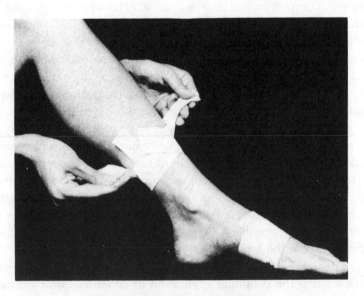

Fig. 12-10. Shin splints strapping.

Patellar tendinitis

The condition of patellar tendon strain is increasing in incidence in the dance field mainly because of the types of static quadriceps contraction activities that are currently practiced; for example, holding a position on half toe with knees bent and the body inclined back. This problem, much like Achilles tendinitis, becomes chronic following just a few acute episodes. The dancer who complains of a constant pain and mild swelling in the area around the patella and who is free from bone spurs or degeneration of the patella most likely will be diagnosed as having patellar tendinitis.

A major cause of patellar tendinitis in dancers is commonly lower leg and thigh malalignment. Normally the patella, which is the largest sesamoid bone and is encased in the quadriceps femoris muslce, is positioned in front of the knee in direct relationship with the intercondylar notch of the femur. In some dancers the patella is out of alignment with this notch and abnormally articulates with the lateral femoral tuberosity, thus wearing away the articular surface of the kneecap and tuberosity. Tendinitis, arthritis, or even chrondro-malacia may occur. Remediation of this problem usually requires avoidance of active dancing and performance of postural exercise with special attention given to the strength of the quadriceps muscle.

Ideally, the dancer with this problem should place the quadriceps muscle at complete rest. If rest is not possible, a therapeutic program of superficial heat and support might prevent further injury. Ultrasound therapy has also been found to be beneficial for chronic problems in this area. A tape support with a spiral elastic wrap often assists the dancer in not exceeding the limits imposed by this problem (Fig. 12-11). Both ice massage and static

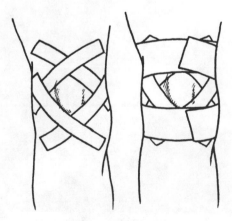

Fig. 12-11. Patella strapping.

stretch have been found to be beneficial in decreasing swelling in some cases. Activities that involve violent static contractions of the quadriceps muscle must be avoided at all costs; however, a slow gradual stretch routing should be initiated before and after an activity session.

"The clicks" (joint noises)

Many dancers complain that when they move, their joints make strange noises similar to clicks, crunches, or thumps. The causes of joint noises are varied. Often the dancer stretches tendons that cross joints to the point that they respond by snapping across the joint when the part is stretched or moved in a certain way. Noises within a joint may also indicate, if associated with some irritation and discomfort, osteophondritis dissecans. In most cases the snapping tendon, if not associated with pain, is not considered harmful, but the dancer should not be encouraged to snap a tendon continually because it may eventually develop into a chronic problem. Also, joint noises can be elicited from a capsule surrounding a joint that becomes slack from continually exceeding automatically normal limits or from within a joint, as in the case of clicks and creaking noises.

13

Sprains, dislocations, and fractures

Although less common than injuries to the musculotendinous unit, injuries to the joint and bone do happen in dance. Sprains, dislocations, and even fractures can result from the rigors of dance. Serious injury occurring to joints or bones results initially from impact forces, with carelessness and fatigue playing a major role. Late in the practice day or just before an opening performance when the dancer is pressing most for perfection seems to be the time when most serious injuries occur. The older the dancer, the more susceptible he or she is to serious joint and bone injuries.

SPRAINS

The most common sprains (Table 12) occurring to the dancer are sprains to the toes, ankles, knees, hip, lower back, and occasionally the wrists. As discussed earlier, the sprain is primarily an injury to the ligamentous supportive structures of a joint. Like contusions and strains, the sprain is categorized into first, second, and third degrees of intensity. The intensity of a sprain is best determined by the extent of the dancer's disability as well as the tenderness elicited by feel or palpation and the amount of hemorrhage and swelling present. Unlike the dancer with a strain or contusion, a dancer with a second-or third-degree sprain must routinely be referred to a physician for X-ray examination and diagnosis, because fracture is commonly associated with a twisted joint. A joint that has lost its ability to function for more than several minutes must be considered to have either a second- or

Table 12. Acute sprain management

Degree of injury	Basic signs	Treatment program				
		Management phase	Physical therapy	Dosage	Reconditioning	Dosage
First degree	Mild twist of joint causing a twinge of discomfort produced by minimal hemorrhage	Step 1: immediate care	1. Apply cold and pressure; 20 min on, 20 min off 2. Elevation 3. Tape or wrap support for continual pressure	24 hr 24 hr Variable	1. Avoid moving joint 2. General sustained exercise	Daily Daily
		Step 2: second day	1. Superficial heat 2. Massage above and below injury, contrast bath 3. Wrap if swelling is present	10 min one to two times daily 5 min one to two times daily	1. Move joint to retain range of movement if pain free	One to two times daily
Second degree	Moderate twist of joint resulting in pain, loss of function for several minutes or longer, and point tenderness; swelling occurs if proper immediate care is not given	Step 1: immediate care	1. Apply cold and pressure; 20 min on, 20 min off 2. Elevation 3. Apply tape or wrap for continual pressure 4. Referral to physician for x-ray examination	48 hr 48 hr 48 hr	1. No weight bearing if ankle or knee 2. Crutch walking 3. General sustained exercise	3 days Daily

	Treatment	Frequency	Exercise	Frequency
Step 2: second or third day	1. Superficial heat (90°)	20 min twice daily	1. No weight bearing if ankle or knee	
	2. Contrast bath	Twice daily	2. Continue crutch walking	
	3. Massage above and below injury	5 min twice daily	3. Move part for range of movement if pain free	Twice daily
	4. Continue wrap for pressure		4. General sustained exercise	Daily
Step 3: third or fourth day	1. Superficial heat (warm—102° F) or contrast baths if swelling is present	Three times daily	1. If ankle or knee, weight bearing with support	
	2. Massage part	Three times daily	2. Move part for range of movement	Twice daily
	3. Analgesic balm packs when generally active	Twice daily	3. General sustained exercise	Twice daily
Step 4	1. Therapy program is continued until dancer is symptom free	Daily	1. Continue until symptom free	Daily

Continued.

Table 12. Acute sprain management—cont'd.

Degree of injury	Basic signs	Treatment program					
		Management phase	Physical therapy	Dosage	Reconditioning	Dosage
Third degree	Severe joint twist causing extreme pain, loss of function over long period, point tenderness, and usually immediate swelling with later discoloration	Step 1: immediate care	1. Cold and pressure 2. Elevation 3. Tape or wrap for constant pressure and stabilization 4. Refer to physician for x-ray examination and medication	48-72 hr 24-48 hr As prescribed	1. No weight bearing if ankle or knee 2. Crutch walking 3. Rest part	3-5 days
		Step 2: third or fourth day	1. Superficial heat (warm) 2. Massage above and below injury 3. Maintain tape or wrap for constant pressure	15 min twice daily 5 min twice daily	1. No weight bearing 2. Crutch walking 3. Move part for range of movement 4. General sustained exercise	 Twice daily Twice daily
		Step 3: fourth or fifth day	1. Superficial heat or contrast bath if swelling persists 2. Massage 3. Analgesic balm pack when active	Three times daily Three times daily	1. Weight bearing if no limp 2. Move part to restore range of movement 3. General sustained exercise	 Twice daily Twice daily
		Step 4	1. Therapy program is continued until dancer is symptom free; support may be required	Daily	1. Continue until symptom free	Daily

third-degree sprain. Ice, pressure, and elevation should be routinely employed to control hemorrhage and swelling in the joint. This procedure is even more important for joint injury than in cases of injury to a muscle, because injured joints rapidly swell with the effusion of blood and serum. A second- or third-degree sprain may demand joint immobilization to ensure a speedy recovery. However, each type of joint injury has its own characteristics in terms of therapeutic requirements. It should also be noted that although a sprain is mainly concerned with ligamentous tissue, it seldom occurs without affecting muscle tendons crossing the joint.

Toe sprain

The barefoot dancer has a high incidence of stubbed toes, particularly the great toe. Jamming against an immovable object and suddenly twisting the great toe are hazards of the dance profession. Usually a sprained toe responds positively to application of the procedures shown in Table 9. However, weight bearing may not be allowed for a time and/or a special strapping may be necessary to provide stability. If the sprain has occurred to toes other than the great toe, the best immobilization procedure is that in which the affected toe is taped to an adjacent unaffected toe.

Great toe strapping (Fig. 13-1). Strapping of the great toe can be initiated by using a combination of 1- and ½-inch tape. The ½-inch tape is started from the middle of the foot, and the tape is carried from the great toe to the first toe, encircling it and then coming over its top and returning to the starting point. Two or three tape strips can be applied and their ends anchored by a 1-inch tape strip encircling the metatarsophalangeal joint. This tape technique supports the second joint of the great toe and the ball of the foot.

Ankle sprain

When considering a sprain, one usually thinks of the ankle joint (Fig. 13-2). Even though structurally the ankle may be considered a moderately strong joint, it is subject to sudden twists, especially when the dancer steps on some irregular surface. The highest incidence of injury is to the outside aspect of the ankle. This occurs when the dancer turns the foot inward, placing an abnormal stretch on the outer ankle ligaments. For the dancer with flat feet and/or pronated feet, inside sprains are more common and more serious in nature. Usually a dancer has a high level of flexibility in the ankle region, and it takes a great deal of force to actually cause a sprain. If this force is great enough, ligaments will be torn and even a part of the outer ankle bone may be pulled away. Also, the center talus bone may roll underneath and strike against the internal ankle bone, causing a fracture on the inside of

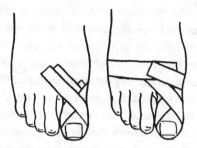

Fig. 13-1. Sprained toe strapping.

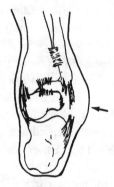

Fig. 13-2. Lateral (outside) ankle sprain.

the ankle. One should note that repeated sprains can lead to an osteoarthritic condition in any joint of the body.

Inability to bear weight on the affected foot and rapid swelling must be considered symptoms of fracture, and a physician should be consulted immediately. Some physicans may routinely apply a cast to a second- or third-degree sprain as well as a fracture for a week or longer to ensure proper repair. On the other hand, some physicans will apply a tape support to the sprain and instruct the dancer to engage in no weight bearing for 2 to 3 days, followed by a program of physical therapy.

The medial, or inside, sprain represents a different problem than the lateral sprain, because even though it occurs less frequently it is more serious than a lateral ankle sprain, because injuring the inside ligaments also affects the inner longitudinal arch. Often dancers who have had medial sprains experience difficulties. It is suggested that, along with regular rehabilitation regimens, the dancer with inside sprain engage in a program of arch and foot conditioning. As in all sprains, once the ligaments of the ankle have been stretched, exercise cannot restore joint stability. Therefore, strapping is the best preventive procedure.

Ankle strapping (Fig. 13-3). The purpose of the ankle strapping technique is to provide mild support to the ankle joint and still allow for foot and ankle mobility. The main materials required are 1- and ½-inch tape and tape adherent. Maintaining the foot in a neutral (90-degree) position, the dancer places an anchor strip about 4 inches above the malleolus and then applies two stirrups along each side of the ankle, starting just in front of the Achilles tendon and overlapping each piece of tape approximately one-half of the width of the preceding piece (Fig. 13-3, A). Once the stirrups are in place, circle strips are applied around the lower leg and down past the malleolus, locking the stirrups in place and providing a mild support to the lower leg tendons (Fig. 13-3, B). Next, two arch strips and a heel lock are applied. The heel lock is applied by starting the tape high on the instep and bringing it behind the ankle, hooking the heel, bringing it under the arch and up on the opposite side, and finishing at the starting point. The tape continues on the opposite side, hooking the heel, crossing the arch, and then returning to the starting point, completing two loops of the heel (Fig. 13-3, C). The purpose of the heel lock is to stabilize the heel and the talus bone.

An additional technique that can be used by itself or in conjunction with ankle strapping is application of an adhesive felt horseshoe (Fig. 13-4). The horseshoe technique can also be used in conjunction with the chronically swollen ankle and the tendons that might be strained in that area. Using ¼-inch adhesive felt, a horseshoe is cut to fit around the outer or medial malleolus.

The use of elastic material in an attempt to support the ankle is discouraged. Yielding elastic cannot adequately stabilize a joint. However, in situations in which there is swelling and the dancer desires to hold another bandage in place, an elastic wrap or tape may be useful.

A good test for the dancer to determine whether an ankle support should be worn is to jump up and down on the affected foot several times. An ankle that has recovered from an injury will usually allow the dancer to spring into the air and support the body on landing.

Knee sprain

The knee joint is made up of many individual joints with articulations between the two femoral condyles, between portions of the knee cartilage (menisci), between the tibia and the knee cartilage, and between the kneecap and thigh bone. All of these individual articulations serve to make the knee

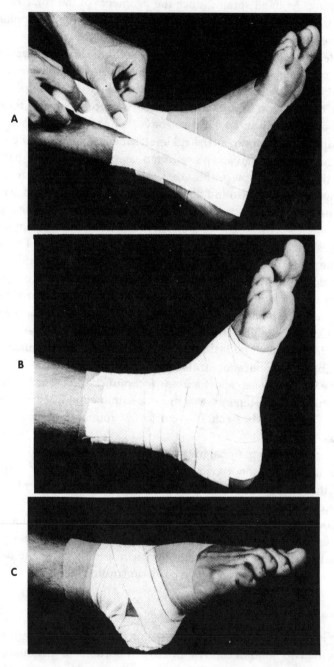

Fig. 13-3. A, Ankle strapping. Applying two stirrups. **B,** Completed ankle strapping without heel lock. **C,** Heel lock alone.

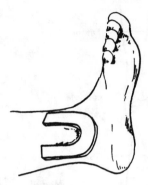

Fig. 13-4. Ankle horseshoe.

one of the most complex joints in the human body (Fig. 13-5). In addition, the knee has a complex system of bursa sacs and a synovial membrane sheath that serves to lubricate the various anatomical structures. This knee cartilage is intended to slightly deepen the joint and to cushion some of the stresses placed on the knee by leaping, running, and other vigorous locomotor activities common to dance. The menisci (knee cartilage) are held loosely on the tibia by ligaments around their outer border. When these ligaments are disrupted and torn, the knee cartilage becomes a loose body within the joint. Stabilizing the knee front to back and back to front are the cruciate ligaments. These ligaments function to prevent the femur from sliding back and forth when the leg is stabilized and, conversely, prevent the leg from sliding back and forth on the femur when it is fixed. Two ligaments provide the knee with side (lateral) stability and are known as the collateral knee ligaments. When the knee is completely straight, the cruciate and both collateral ligaments are right. Also, in the last few degrees of leg straightening, the knee initiates a screwing down by externally rotating. In a semiflexed position, the cruciates loosen along with the lateral collateral ligaments so that the primary stabilizing element of the knee becomes the medial collateral ligament.

In dance, the sprained knee occurs much less often than the strain; however, under adverse conditions the dancer can acquire a severely sprained knee. The primary cause of knee sprain in dance from the sudden torsion, or twisting, of the body with the affected leg planted or fixed to the floor. Under these circumstances both the collateral ligaments and the cruciates could be affected if the knee is slightly flexed. It is not typical for a single acute traumatic situation to cause a knee sprain; instead, repeated torsion injuries to the knee gradually cause a general laxity in all of the supporting ligaments, making the knee increasingly vulnerable to injury.

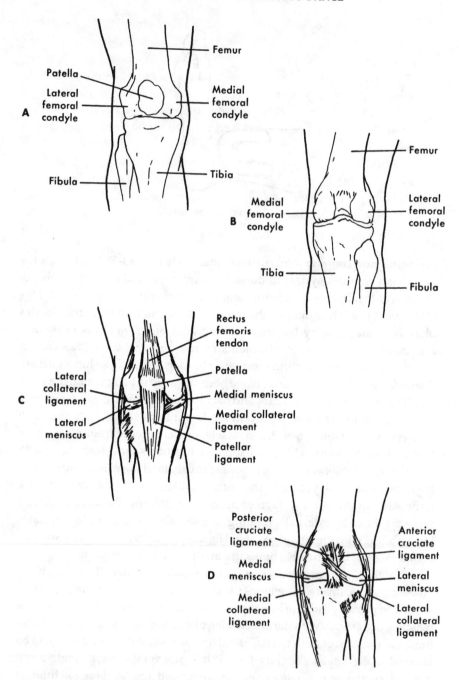

Fig. 13-5. Knee anatomy: **A**, front view; **B**, back view. Knee ligaments: **C**, front view; **D**, back view.

A controversional factor in the causation of knee injury is the deep knee bend. Some authorities say that the deep knee bend should be avoided at all costs because it tends to stretch the internal cruciate ligaments, producing an unstable knee. This is particularly true when deep knee bends are initiated along with supporting heavy weight or when the dancer has bulky legs that force open the knee joint when in a full squat position. I believe that full flexion of the knee is normal and can be initiated safely if performed under controlled conditions. Therefore, the dancer is cautioned against sudden uncontrolled ballistic squats that tend to open up the knee joint suddenly, tearing its internal supporting ligaments. Plies should also be executed under controlled conditions with the thigh, leg, ankle, and foot maintained in good alignment. The dancer who, from a demi-plie, suddenly extends the legs into a jump places great rotary stress on the knee from the screwing down action of the lower leg.

The teacher of dance should realize that different body builds coupled with a given set of situations can make the dancer more or less prone to knee injury. For example, a poorly conditioned dancer may not have the muscle control to prevent bouncing on the knees in a squat position; therefore, until conditioning is appropriate, grand plies should be postponed. Also, the dancer who is short-limbed and stocky or has heavy thighs may be more prone to knee injury than the long, lanky person; in the grand plie position the bulky thigh tends to bulge, causing the knee joint to be adversely forced open. The degree of knee sprain is often difficult to assess accurately. The best time to determine the extent of any injury is immediately after it occurs. The longer the period before assessment, the less accurate will be its determination. Because of the complexity of the knee, the extent of pathological damage is often masked by rapid swelling. Making a completely accurate examination after 24 hours is almost impossible.

Evaluation is first made by observing the dancer's ability to support body weight on the affected leg. Often when the knee is seriously injured the dancer is unable to place the foot flat on the floor and is forced to walk on the toes of the injured leg. Observation may also detect very rapid swelling in and about the knee joint. A second factor in determining the extent of a knee sprain is by palpating for tender areas. First, the soft musculature is felt, and then the bone, capsular, and ligamentous tissue is felt. If tenderness is found on palpation of capsular and ligamentous tissue, one might conclude that the knee support structures have been affected. The next factor in determining the seriousness of a knee sprain is to assess the extent of abnormal mobility present. This must be done before effusion (fluid accumulation) has occurred in the knee to mask the injury. Laxity in either of the collateral ligaments will be demonstrated by abnormal movement in a lateral or medial direction. Laxity in the cruciate ligament will display an anterior or posterior instability.

It is of the utmost importance that cold, compression by an elastic wrap, and elevation be applied immediately to the sprained knee. In addition to the general management procedures listed in Table 12, the dancer should engage in a program of immediate knee strength maintenance. The quadriceps muscles, the main extensor muscles of the knee, atrophy faster than almost any muscle in the body when not used. To prevent this problem, the dancer should immediately engage in a program of reconditioning. While the knee is being treated with cold, pressure, and elevation, the dancer should engage in muscle setting, which includes statically contracting and relaxing the quadriceps muscles with the knee kept in a fully extended position. Muscle setting maintains stimulation to the quadriceps muscle and helps decrease atrophy. At no time, however, should the injured knee be flexed and extended in the initial acute stage; it should be kept in a fully extended position. After quadriceps setting, the dancer can progress into reconditioning exercises by executing straight leg raises from the front lying position and back lying position as well as brushes (tendu). The dancer must always remember not to bend the knee until the acute symptoms have been overcome. Following the acute stage the dancer can engage in a graduated program of knee flexion and extension, gradually regaining a full range of joint movement. Once range of movement exercises have begun, a program of progressive resistance exercises can begin, using only very light resistance at first.

The dancer is ready to return to full dance activity when the knee has redeveloped its strength and full range of movement and can withstand the stresses of lateral body movements without pain or instability.

Often a tape support is beneficial in the later stages of a knee sprain. Tape support is much preferred to elastic wraps and braces, which for the most part do not provide sufficient stabilization. Because the dancer needs complete knee mobility, it is extremely difficult to apply tape that will allow adequate movement and provide stabilization at the same time. Two techniques of strapping are presented; they can be added to or modified, depending on individual needs.

Technique A: knee X strapping (Fig. 13-6). This technique is designed to assist the dancer when there is lateral or medial instability. The tape is applied in a pattern executed on both sides of the knee. However, in a dance situation this may drastically restrict knee mobility, and therefore only the affected side should be taped. The primary materials needed are 2-inch linen tape, 3-inch elastic tape, and skin adherent. A circular 2-inch linen tape strip is placed as an anchor around the thigh approximately 8 to 10 inches above the patella and around the center of the calf. These anchor strips should be

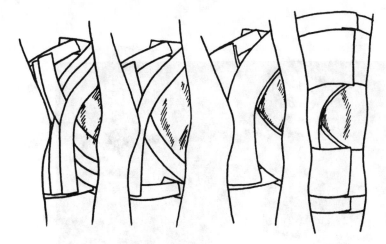

Fig. 13-6. Knee X strapping.

applied loosely; they can be very restricting as the muscle expands from being engorged with blood. An X pattern is applied to the area over the sprain. If both sides of the knee are to be taped, the X's would be initiated in an alternate pattern. Each X should be started behind the medial condyle from the lower anchor strip and be carried upward, attaching to the thigh anchor strip. A series of three X's is applied. However, the dancer should be cautious not to restrict the kneecap, mainly because the patella must be unrestricted if the knee is to bend. The X strips nearest the bend of the kneecap should be tucked under about ¼ inch along their outer border to protect the top from tear. Once the linen tape is in place a 3-inch elastic strip is applied over the X. The tape is locked in place by encircling the thigh and calf with elastic tape strips. If elastic tape is not available to the dancer, an elastic wrap can be applied with a spiral technique over the linen tape to ensure that the tape does not loosen.

Technique B: rotary knee strapping (Fig. 13-7). Rotary knee strapping is designed for knee torsion injuries. Materials needed are 3-inch elastic tape, skin adherent, and a 4-inch pad. As in technique A, the knee is bent approximately 15 degrees. A 10-inch piece of elastic tape is cut and nipped at both ends and torn about 4 inches from its center. A gauze pad is placed behind the knee, and the 4-inch center of the torn elastic tape is placed directly over the gauze pad. The torn ends of the elastic tape strip are pulled taut, overlapping in front of the knee on either side of the patella. The second phase starts at the middle of the gastrocnemius with the application of a 3-inch elastic tape strip.

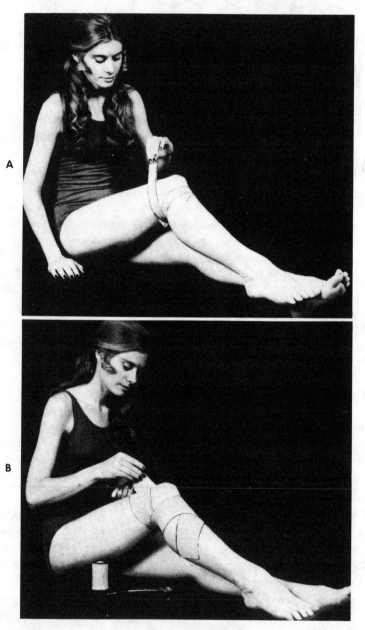

Fig. 13-7. Rotary knee strapping. **A,** Phase 1. **B,** Phase 2.

The tape is brought to the front of the leg and then directly behind the knee, ending in front of the thigh. Only one strip should be applied in cases where the dancer requires a great deal of mobility. If a great deal of knee instability is present, the spiral strips can be retraced with additional strips of elastic tape. Once in place, the spirals are locked with elastic strips around both the thigh and calf.

Hip sprain

Because the hip joint is the strongest and one of the best protected joints in the body, it seldom is sprained. However, even though the hip joint is made up of well-supported bone, ligaments, and muscles, it can be sprained if it is put suddenly in a abnormal position. Sprain of the hip joint most often occurs when the foot of the dancer is firmly planted on the floor and the trunk is suddenly forced into an awkward or opposing direction. The most obvious sign of a sprain is inability to move the thigh in a circular motion. A dancer who warms up properly and stretches the hip in all directions seldom incurs a sprain. However, the dancer is most prone to chronic sprains of the hip in which the supporting capsule and ligaments are overstretched for a long period. Under these conditions, the capsule and ligaments become unable to maintain the head of the femur firmly in the hip socket, and the dancer often complains of the hip feeling like it goes in and out of place when placed in a particular position.

The depth of the tissue surrounding the hip joint makes physical therapy difficult to administer. Rest of the injured hip joint gives the most positive reward. When symptoms of sprain have significantly subsided, a program of gradual stretching can be started. However, it is important that the hip region regain tone and strength of all the major muscles in that area. A strength program is necessary, because ligamentous tissue once stretched can only be tightened by surgical intervention; therefore, muscle strength must then replace these supporting structures.

Lower back sprain

The lower back injury was discussed at some length in Chapter 12; however, in this section the deeper injuries will be discussed. As in many body regions, it is often difficult to ascertain if an injury is muscular or involves the deeper joint structures or both. This is particularly true in the lower back region. There are many terms that describe a lower back condition, most of which are misleading or too general to really pinpoint the exact nature of a condition. These expressions are sciatica, lumbosacral sprains, and sacroiliac sprains.

Most injuries to the lower back region are the result of repeated acute injuries, not just one episode of a sudden twist or extension movement. The structurally deformed or muscularly weak lower back is highly susceptible to stress and pathological damage.

A *radiating pain* down the leg when the back is moved can be caused by several different factors as discussed in Chapter 12. A pain that radiates down the leg to the knee may be the result of pressure on the large sciatic nerve or impingement on nerves in the lumbar region. Dancers should seek professional help if they have a backache with radiating pain, numbness, and/or a tingling sensation.

Repeated trauma to the lower back can eventually result in a herniated disc. The tendency toward this problem can be increased by degeneration of a disc that has become narrow from repeated stresses and abnormal tensions in that area. A movement that suddenly increases the pressure of the internal viscous material (the nucleus pulposus) located in the center of the disc that has become narrow from repeated stresses and abnormal tensions in that area. A movement that suddenly increases the pressure of the internal viscous material (the nucleus pulposus) located in the center of the disc may force a rupturing and spilling of this material outside the vertebrae, placing painful pressure on spinal nerves. The gnawing and chronically painful lower back may be caused by a herniated disc. A dancer with lower back pain that fails to respond to normal physical therapy should be referred to a physician; the herniated disc often requires surgery. In almost every case, lower back sprain must be treated as a chronic problem that responds best to the conservative treatment of rest, sleeping on a firm surface or water bed, superficial and deep heat, and mild stretching. In cases of lower back problems, the strengthening of abdominal muscles and stretching of the lower back and hip flexors must be considered in addition to realigning the pelvis if lordosis is present.

A good exercise for strengthening the lower back is for the dancer to lie on the back on a flat surface with knees bent up. The dancer rolls the pelvis forward, flattening the lower back. While this position is held, the pelvis is raised from the table 2 to 3 inches and held for a count of 10.

DISLOCATIONS

Dislocations (Table 10) are mentioned briefly here because they belong in the category of the most severe joint sprains. Although uncommon in dance, complete dislocation, or luxation, means that there is a complete disassociation of the body parts that make up a joint. More common, however, is partial dislocation, or subluxation, which is often described by the dancer

Table 13. Chronic joint injury management

Common conditions	Basic signs	Management phase	Treatment program				
			Physical therapy	Dosage	Reconditioning	Dosage
Recurrent dislocation, arthritis, and osteochondritis	Continuous low-grade inflammation in and around joint producing constant pain on movement, local weakness, and swelling	Symptomatic	1. Superficial heat	Three times daily	1. Rest of part	
			2. Analgesic balm	Three times daily	2. Movement of part to maintain range of movement	Three times daily
			3. Massage	Three times daily	3. General sustained exercise	Twice daily
			4. Deep heat	Three times daily		

Adapted from Klafs, C. E., and Arnheim, D. D.: Modern principles of athletic training, ed. 4, St. Louis, 1977, The C. V. Mosby Co.

as "I felt it go out and then it seemed to snap back in." In dance the serious toe stub can result in a dislocation; falling on the outstretched hand can cause the fingers to become dislocated.

However, the most common dislocation in dance, with the highest incidence occurring among female dancers, is the kneecap that "goes out of place." Individuals with poor quadriceps muscle tone or those with a shallow recess for the patella to glide on and poor leg alignment seem to be susceptible to this problem. The increased angle of pull of the quadriceps tendon as a result of the wider hip has been suggested as the reason females have a higher incidence of patella dislocation than males. This problem, coupled with a congenital flattening of the lateral femoral condyle where the patella is recessed, increases the possibility of dislocating the kneecap. The right circumstance (such as having the patella knocked or hit by another dancer when the quadriceps is relaxed) can cause the patella to slide over and become lodged on the lateral aspect of the knee. For example, not turning the knee out and over the foot on the first step of a triplet turn (the plie) can force the kneecap to be pulled laterally. In this situation the dancer is unable to move the leg and is caught with the knee in a semiflexed position. It is obvious that this situation is a medical problem, but ice and pressure should still be applied to control the hemorrhage until a physician can give treatment. Following reduction of this dislocation, a cast or rigid bandage may be applied for 2 or 3 weeks.

It is also true that dancers complain that they feel their hip "go out" when they move in a particular way. This is particularly true for those who have overstretched the hip joint ligament and capsule. It is important that the dancer who has a loose hip problem avoid extreme stretching movements that cause the hip joint to be continually subluxated; this can eventually result in degeneration and a subsequent osteoarthritic problem. For dancers with chronically dislocating hips, it is suggested that they engage in a vigorous muscle conditioning program and avoid hip stretching until there is extremely good muscle tone and control in that area.

JOINT DEGENERATION

Sometimes occurring to the dancer's joints, particularly those of the hip and knee, joint degeneration (Table 13) is a condition that results in a softening of the articular surfaces. This degenerative condition seems to be more apparent in late childhood and early adolescence, but the results of this problem can be carried over into adulthood and even old age. Because of the softening of the articular surface (chondromalasia), pieces of material are sloughed off into the joint (osteochondritis dissecans), often getting caught during movement and making the so-called creaking noises. Loose bodies in a joint are commonly called "joint mice." This type of degeneration can react with pain, swelling, and other signs of general inflammation. Teachers of dance should refer any student with these symptoms to a physician. The treatment of choice is often rest with decreasing amounts of weight bearing until nature has been allowed to resolve the problem.

FRACTURES

Although fractures that occur as a result of being hit are rare in dance, the fracture does occur as a result of a sudden twist or chronic stress. As mentioned earlier, fractures can be associated with a severe wrenching of a joint and a sudden pulling of muscle in which bone is pulled away. More commonly, fractures occur in dance because of chronic fatigue in a particular body part, causing agonist and antagonist muscles to pull at the same time, which produces a shearing action on a particular bone. In this situation the spontaneous, or stress, fracture occurs. Stress fractures occur by accumulated impact and rhythmic shock to an area where muscles are not directly associated. The most common sites for stress fractures in dancers are the metatarsal region of the foot, the fibula, and less commonly, the tibia. This spontaneous fracture can be prevented when shock is absorbed by proper shoes and more resilient stage surfaces. The dancer should always be encouraged to refer to a physician any injury that fails to respond to first aid and palliative treatment.

Epilogue

The demands of dance on the human body can be highly beneficial or may become deleterious, depending on the nature of the dance form, the state of the dancer's body, and/or the environment in which the dancer performs. The dancer and the teacher of dance must be aware of the limits of the human body and be able to impart the best injury prevention methods available. The dancer must develop an internal awareness of what is a reasonable stress for the body to tolerate and differentiate between pain that indicates the outcome of hard work and pain that is pathological. Early injury recognition and appropriate immediate and follow-up care are crucial to effective injury management.

References

1. Abraham, W.M.: Factors in delayed muscle soreness, Med. Sci. Sports 9(1):11–20, 1977.
2. Alfred, R.H., and Bergfeld, J.A.: Diagnosis and Management of Stress Fractures of the Foot, The Phys. and Sportsmed. 15(8):83–89, Aug. 1987.
3. Arnheim, D.D.: Modern principles of athletic training, St. Louis: Times Mirror/Mosby College Publishing, 1987.
4. Bachrach, R.M.: Injuries to the Dancer's Spine, in Ryan, A.J., and Stephens, R.E. Dance medicine: a comprehensive guide, Chicago: Pluribus Press, 1987.
5. Belyea, C.: "Ta'i chi ch'uan," in Hill, A., ed., A visual encyclopedia of unconventional medicine, New York: Crown Publishers, Inc., 1979.
6. Benson, J.E., and others: Nutritional considerations for ballet dancers, in Clarkson, P.M., and Skrinar, M. Science of dance training, Champaign, Illinois: Human Kinetics Books, 1988.
7. Breen, A.C.: Chiropractice, in Hill, A. ed., A visual encyclopedia of unconventional medicine, New York: Crown Publishers, Inc., 1979.
8. Braisted, J.R., and others: The adolescent ballet dancer: nutritional practices and characteristics associated with anorexia nervosa, Journal of Adolescent Health Care 6:365–371, Sept. 1985.
9. Brooks, Gunn, and others: The relation of eating problems and ammenorrhea in ballet dancers, Medicine Science Sports Exercise 19:41–44, Feb. 1987.
10. DeLorme, T.L., and Watkins, A.L.: Progressive resistance exercise. New York: Appleton-Century-Crofts, 1951.
11. Fitt, S.F.: Dance kinesiology, New York: Schirmer Books, 1988.
12. Humphrey, D.: The art of making dances, New York: Rinehart and Co., Inc., 1959; Princeton, NJ: Princeton Book Company, Publishers, 1990.
13. Jacobs, M., and Young, R.: Snapping hip phenonemon among dancers, Am. Correct. Ther. J. 32(3):92–97, May-June, 1978.
14. Klafs, C.D., and Lyon, M.L.: The female athlete, ed. 2, St. Louis: The C.V. Mosby Co., 1978.

15. Knott, M., and Voss, D.E.: Proprioceptive neuromuscular facilitation, ed. 2, New York: Harper & Row, Publishers, Inc., 1968.
16. Lesio, L.: Toward Efficient Alignment, Journal of Physical Education, Recreation and Dance 57(4):73–76, April 1986.
17. Myers, M.: What dance medicine and science mean to the dancer, in Clarkson, P.M., and Skrinar, M. Science of Dance Training, Champaign, Ill.: Human Kinetics Books, 1988.
18. Neil-Rose, S.: Acupuncture, in Hill, A. ed., A visual encyclopedia of unconventional medicine, New York: Crown Publishers, Inc., 1979.
19. Ryan, A.J., and Stephens, R.E.: The Epidemiology of Dance Injuries, in Ryan, A.J., and Stephens, R.E. Dance medicine: a comprehensive guide, Chicago: Pluribus Press, 1987.
20. Ryan, A.J.: What is dance medicine? A physician's perspective, in Clarkson, P.M., and Skrinar, M. Science of dance training, Champaign, Ill. Human Kinetics Books, 1988.
21. Ryan, A.J., and others: Injuries of ballet dancers. The Phys. and Sportsmed. 4:43–57, Nov. 1976.
22. Seals, J.: Dance Surfaces, in Ryan, A.J., and Stephens, R.E. Dance medicine: a comprehensive guide, Chicago: Pluribus Press, 1987.
23. Stephens, R.E.: The etiology of injuries in ballet, in Ryan, A.J., and Stephens, R.E. Dance medicine: a comprehensive guide, Chicago: Pluribus Press, 1987.
24. Tara, W.: Shiatsu, in Hill, A. ed., A visual encyclopedia of unconventional medicine, New York: Crown Publishers, Inc., 1979.
25. Washington, E.L.: Musculoskeletal Problems in Modern, Jazz and "Show Biz" Dancers, in Ryan, A.J., and Stephens, R.E. Dance medicine: a comprehensive guide. Chicago: Pluribus Press, 1987.
26. Welch, P.K., and others: Nutrition education, body composition, and dietary intake of female college athletes, The Phys. and Sports Med., 15(1):63–74, Jan. 1987.

Glossary

abduction Movement of a part away from the midline of the body (opposite of adduction).

abrasion Superficial wound of the skin resulting from friction or the scraping of the skin against a hard surface such as the floor.

acute Sharp, abrupt, sudden, such as acute pain; there is a quick onset and the course is usually short in duration.

adduction Movement of a part toward the midline of the body (opposite of abduction).

agonist muscle The muscle or muscle group that is acting or contracting.

antagonist muscle The muscle or muscle group that is in opposition to the agonist (contracting) muscle.

anterior Situated in front of or in the forward part.

arm backward extension Backward movement of the arm at the shoulder from a neutral starting position at the side of the body.

articulation Place at which bones meet to form a joint.

avlusion Tearing or pulling away of a part of a structure.

ballistic stretch Bouncing stretch.

basketweave Method of strapping by interweaving tape to provide extra strength.

bursa Small closed sac that is lined with specialized connective tissue and contains synovial fluid; usually located over bony prominences where muscles or tendons glide.

cartilage Specialized form of connective tissue with varying amounts of intercellular matrix that is nonvascular and found in various parts of the body.

charley horse Contusion of quadriceps muscle characterized by pain and swelling produced by intramuscular bleeding.

chronic Marked by long duration; continued; not acute; may also refer to a recurrent injury or one that has not responded to treatment.

contusion Bruise of superficial or deep body tissues without a break in the covering of the skin; caused by external force.

counterirritant Agent that is applied to the skin surface to produce a mild irritation and an analgesic effect.

dislocation Either a partial or complete displacement of a bone from its normal position in a joint.

ecchymosis Collection of blood under the skin (black and blue color).

epiphysis That part of a bone that is concerned with growth in length (for example, the ends of the long bones).

eversion Turning the sole of the foot outward, away from the midline of the body.

extension Returning to a starting position in a hinge joint such as the elbow or knee; stretching a limb outward (opposite of flexion).

fascia Fibrous membrane that covers, supports, and separates muscles.

flexion Movement away from extension in a hinge joint such as the elbow or knee; a bending movement (opposite of extension).

fracture Broken bone.

genu recurvatum Hyperextension of the knee joint.

genu valgum Knock-knee.

genu varum Bowleg.

gradual stretch Stretching the musculotendinous unit by assuming a position in which the muscle is stretched gradually (opposite of ballistic stretch).

hamstring muscles Muscles in the back of the thigh (biceps femoris, semitendinosus, and semimembranosus) that extent the thigh and flex the leg at the knee.

heel lock Process of stabilizing the heel with tape or a wrap.

hematoma Circumscribed collection of blood in a muscle following trauma.

hot spot Hot or irritated feeling on the foot that occurs just before a friction blister.

inflammation Reaction of tissues to an injury or infection; characterized by heat, swelling, redness, pain, and sometimes loss of function.

inversion Turning of the sole of the foot inward, toward the midline of the body.

isometric Form of muscular contraction in which the muscle length does not change.

isotonic Form of muscular contraction in which the muscle length changes.

laceration Skin tear having jagged edges.

lateral On the outer side, as distinguished from the medial (inner) side.

ligament Band of fibrous connective tissue that stabilizes joints.

lumbosacral Concerning the area of the back where the lumbar and sacral areas are in contact.

luxation Complete dislocation.

medial On the middle or inner side, as compared with the later (outer) side.

meniscus Semilunar cartilage of the knee joint.

muscle stretch facilitation Muscle relaxation through inhibition of antagonist muscle to increase a muscle stretch.

pinched nerve Compression of a nerve root causing a contusion of the root.

plantar Referring to the sole of the foot.

posterior Behind or in back of.

reduction Return to a normal position, as in reduction of a dislocated shoulder.

rubefacient Substance that causes the skin to redden when applied topically.

scoliosis Lateral curvature of the spine.

shin splints Painful and disabling condition of the lower leg that results from a muscle strain.

spasm Involuntary contraction of one or more muscles.

sprain Injury of the supporting ligaments and other tissue associated with a joint following and as a result of a sudden twist.

static stretch Gradual stretch.

strapping (tapping) Use of adhesive tape to support or protect a joint.

subluxation Partial or incomplete dislocation.

tendinitis Irritation, inflammation, and swelling of a tendon.

tendon Band of fibrous connective tissue that forms the end of a muscle and inserts into a bone controlling the direction of muscle pull.

tenosynovitis Inflammation of the tendon sheath.

Index